it ain't over 'til the *thin* lady sings

Who Is Your Inner "Thin Lady"?*

You do have one, you know
It's the part of you that feels good in your body
Loves to run just for the joy of it
Knows how to dance and move and play

Your inner Thin Lady
Walks down the street with head held high
Unashamed, confident, happy
Not worried about how she looks
Because her life is already full
Of love and realized dreams

Why not let her come out?
Why not realize your dreams?
It is possible!
The answer is within

* *To my male readers:* Yes, you have an inner thin person, too!

D1115799

*This book is dedicated
to my loving friends and family members,
and to those who are dealing
with food and body-image issues.*

*May we all keep on loving our way
into healthier and happier lives.*

Ordering
Trade bookstores in the U.S. and Canada please contact:

Publishers Group West
1700 Fourth Street, Berkeley CA 94710
Phone: (800) 788-3123   Fax: (510) 528-3444

Hunter House books are available at bulk discounts for textbook course
adoptions; to qualifying community, health-care, and government
organizations; and for special promotions and fund-raising.
For details please contact:

Special Sales Department
Hunter House Inc., PO Box 2914, Alameda CA 94501-0914
Phone: (510) 865-5282   Fax: (510) 865-4295
E-mail: ordering@hunterhouse.com

Individuals can order our books from most bookstores,
by calling **(800) 266-5592**, or from our website at
www.hunterhouse.com

it ain't **over**
'til the
thin lady
sings

How to Make Your
Weight Loss Surgery
a Lasting Success

Michelle Ritchie, CSAC, ICRC

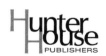

Hunter
House
PUBLISHERS

Hunter House Inc., Publishers
PO Box 2914
Alameda CA   94501-0914

Library of Congress Cataloging-in-Publication Data
Ritchie, Michelle.
It ain't over 'til the thin lady sings : making your weight loss surgery
a lasting success / Michelle Ritchie. — 1st ed.
p.   cm.
Includes index.
ISBN-13: 978-0-89793-491-6 (pbk.)
ISBN-10: 0-89793-491-1 (pbk.)
1. Obesity—Surgery. I. Title.
RD540.R58 2007
617.4'3—dc22   2007017304

Project Credits

Cover Design	Brian Dittmar Graphic Design
Book Production	John McKercher
Developmental and Copy Editor	Kelley Blewster
Proofreader	John David Marion
Indexers	Robert and Cynthia Swanson
Acquisitions Editor	Jeanne Brondino
Editor	Alexandra Mummery
Senior Marketing Associate	Reina Santana
Rights Coordinator	Candace Groskreutz
Interns	Amy Hagelin, Alexi Ueltzen, Julia Wang
Customer Service Manager	Christina Sverdrup
Order Fulfillment	Washul Lakdhon
Administrator	Theresa Nelson
Computer Support	Peter Eichelberger
Publisher	Kiran S. Rana

Printed and Bound by Bang Printing, Brainerd, Minnesota

Manufactured in the United States of America

9 8 7 6 5 4 3 2 1   First Edition   07 08 09 10 11

Contents

To My Readers

The book you're about to read offers information on the pros and cons of weight loss surgery and discusses the "before, during, and after" aspects of the procedure. Weight loss surgery has been an effective tool for me and for many others, but I must emphasize to you that *there are some significant health risks associated with this kind of procedure.* These may include digestive concerns ranging from short-term, mild symptoms that resolve quickly to more serious problems that may result in malnutrition, excessive weight loss, anemia, and/or permanent digestive discomfort. The average mortality rate from weight loss surgery is approximately one in two hundred. Consulting with your physician and with other health-care professionals specific to your needs is a must before deciding to undergo weight loss surgery. Consider their advice carefully in making your decision.

Because of the potential health risks, I am *not* promoting weight loss surgery as an antidote to overeating or as a cure for food addiction. Instead, I strongly encourage anyone who has had chronic weight problems to try any and all healthy alternatives to surgery, such as good nutrition, consistent exercise, counseling, support groups, and the like, before seriously considering surgery. In fact, much of this book is devoted to describing many such healthy alternatives. It offers a "buffet" of support methods for body, mind, heart, and spirit, some of which will be new to you. You'll be surprised by how effective they are.

I highly recommend giving your best effort to these healthy alternatives before committing yourself to weight loss surgery. Whether you end up choosing surgery or not, in the long run these tools will give you a solid, lasting foundation for mind, heart, and spirit—a foundation that surgery alone cannot provide. They will help you create enjoyable lifestyle changes, ones that will work not just for weight loss surgery patients, but also for anyone who wants to become their healthiest and best self!

For a more comprehensive look at the potential complications of weight loss surgery and the most recent statistics on how often they occur, please consult the websites and books recoommended in the Resources section located at the back of this book.

Important Note

The material in this book is intended to provide a review of information regarding weight loss surgery. Every effort has been made to provide accurate and dependable information. The contents of this book have been compiled through professional research and in consultation with medical and mental-health professionals. However, health-care professionals have differing opinions, and advances in medical and scientific research are made very quickly, so some of the information may become outdated.

Therefore, the publisher, authors, and editors, as well as the professionals quoted in the book, cannot be held responsible for any error, omission, or dated material. The authors and publisher assume no responsibility for any outcome of applying the information in this book in a program of self-care or under the care of a licensed practitioner. If you have questions concerning your nutrition or diet, or about the application of the information described in this book, consult a qualified health-care professional.

The true stories of weight loss surgery patients and others that are included in this book have been printed with their permission. Some individuals chose to share their stories but remain anonymous, and in these cases all identifying data have been changed to protect their privacy. The author wishes to express her gratitude and appreciation to all those who shared their stories.

Foreword

Several years ago, when I wished to refer a severely overweight patient of mine for bariatric (weight loss) surgery, our surgeon informed me that he'd stopped performing these procedures because "the postoperative patients had problems following their aftercare plan, since they had no support after surgery." He said that they needed emotional, nutritional, and medical support that was far beyond the scope of his practice, and without it they often failed. But my patient Tina, a thirty-eight-year-old single mother, was at the point where she needed to lose the weight or end up in a wheelchair. So I promised the surgeon that I would personally support her. She underwent the procedure shortly thereafter with no major complications.

A few weeks later I joined Tina and four other post-op weight loss surgery (WLS) patients for their first support group meeting. Together we formed the nucleus of a support group that was to change all our lives and change our health-care institution forever. We created a model for the comprehensive care of WLS patients, working to develop an educational and psychological safety net that would support true lifestyle changes over the long haul, not just provide a surgical "magic pill." I am fortunate to work with a dedicated and caring team of surgeons, behaviorists, pharmacists, nurses, nutritionists, and physical therapists. Together we shepherd patients through an intensive screening process before approving them for surgery, and we follow them postoperatively over the long term. I travel the nation speaking to clinics and hospitals about our support program, which has become a role model when it comes to this kind of surgery.

The public knows very little about weight loss surgery—and what they do know is often full of exaggeration and misinformation. This frequently includes seeing weight loss surgery as a "quick fix," requiring no effort on the part of the patient. However, nothing could be further from the truth. Although the average bariatric patient does initially lose 50 to 80 percent of their excess body weight during the first year post-op, after that they can return to nearly normal eating patterns and become just as susceptible as the average person to gaining the weight back again. Theirs is a lifetime struggle.

I have been lucky to meet grand souls such as Michelle Ritchie along the way. Her book is exceptional for many reasons. First, it is written by an "average Jane," if you will, who nevertheless has a dramatic life history that touches on many commonalties of our severely obese population. Furthermore, in relating Michelle's journey, the book takes us from the preoperative patient's concerns through the fifth postoperative year. Michelle's book is a critical contribution to our understanding of the effects of severe obesity and of the physical and psychological changes that occur when someone loses over a hundred pounds within a relatively short period of time.

I also appreciate Michelle's take on the "eat healthy for life" nutrition and exercise plan, and I applaud her comprehensive look at all the areas that affect people who overeat—not just their diet, but the body-mind-spirit connection. Understanding that connection is the key to maintaining weight loss over the long haul, not just for the gastric bypass patient, but for anyone.

I know that Michelle's book will be a helpful tool to those considering surgery and will provide support for those who are still working on their health postoperatively. While weight loss surgery is not, and should not be, for everyone, for those who choose this path it can be a lifesaving transformation, as you will discover in this book.

— Sasha Stiles, M.D., MPH

Dr. Stiles is the medical director for Kaiser Permanente's Bariatric Surgery Division and the medical director for the Kaiser Permanente Care Management Institute. In addition to being a physician, she also holds a master's degree in public health and is a member of the American Society of Bariatric Surgery. She travels the country speaking about the rights of obese patients and spearheading advancements in the medical interventions available to them.

Acknowledgments

My deepest gratitude to the bariatric team at Kaiser Permanente Hawaii—you gave me a new life with this surgery, and all your wonderful support helped me to realize this book.

Much appreciation to my dear friends and loved ones—I couldn't do it without your support and occasional kick in the.... Well, thanks for your help! Gratitude to Eve, Margaret, Dianne, Torrie, Eric, Anoai, and more.

And to all the wonderful, fun, cool baristas at Starbucks Maui, who encouraged me, bugged me, and kept me fueled up to the finish line— you guys were great!

I hope my story will offer encouragement and inspiration to those who come after me—just as all of you motivated and inspired me to reach for my highest and best self.

Introduction

Out of the
Frying Pan and
into the...
Volcano?

Haleakala, Maui, Hawaii

Inside the volcano, the afternoon sun was fading fast. Golden light turned chill gray as the mist rose around us, curling out from behind jagged lava crags, veiling the path. The crunch of our boots on the cinder trail made the only sound in the deep silence, as we hurried toward the cabin that was barely visible in the distance.

We were inside Haleakala crater, an extinct volcano atop the island of Maui. The valley within this crater is seven miles long, larger than the island of Manhattan. It has its own ecosystem and contains unique flora and fauna found nowhere else on Earth. It even has its own weather, which can range from rainbow-filled sunshine to brief but violent storms, sometimes shifting from one to the other extreme within minutes.

We're hiking to Kaupo Gap, a beautiful, nearly inaccessible site located at the farthest point inside the crater. People who have made this pilgrimage talk about twisted limbs, lost toenails, and hypothermia as if they were badges of honor.

Maybe they are.

You won't find your way here on any casual stroll. The trail zigzags down from the highest point on Maui, at over ten thousand feet, all the way down to sea level. You have to train for this trek, bring plenty of water and good shoes, and even then, most people suffer some sort of injury. It's dangerously beautiful; on their return home, dirty and exhausted but somehow radiant, survivors report that it's grueling but worth it.

Many thousands of sightseers have traveled the first quarter mile of this trail, or just looked out over the rim and snapped a photo, so they could say they'd been there.

None of them had the privilege of entering the place where we now stood.

I realized I was somewhere very special, somewhere that few people have ever seen, or will ever get to see. The only way to get here is to walk it—all twenty-one rocky miles of it. It doesn't matter if you're rich or powerful—no helicopter will drop you here and no limousine can carry you in style. You have to be strong enough, brave enough, and motivated enough to push through your tiredness, your little aches and pains, to obtain this reward.

Not many people can do it, really.

But I just did.

I just did!

Because for the first time in my life, I could.

I tell you this story because it exemplifies so much of what my life is about today. I can be like the tourist and look at life from the rim, or I can jump in and "trudge the road of happy destiny," as the AA book says. Most of the time, I jump!

Nowadays, I've learned to practice all the tools I teach others about how to deal successfully with food, eating, and body image. I'm aware of what I'm feeling before the old knee-jerk reaction sets in, before I go for the food to "fix" an uncomfortable moment. I can take that moment of clarity to choose a different path and find a way to truly nurture myself. Most of the time I will call a friend, or write in my journal, or go for a walk, or pray. Some of the time, I still eat when that's not the best choice.

I met my first WLS (weight loss surgery) patient online in the fall of 2001 as I was searching the Internet for information about the procedure. Sharon quickly became an e-mail friend, and she generously offered her time and support while I asked a million questions about the surgery.

When we met in person a few weeks later, I was a little shocked. Though she'd had her surgery a few years before, she still weighed 245 pounds, not exactly slender. When I hesitantly asked her if she was satisfied with the results of the surgery, she sighed and said, "Well, I started out at nearly four hundred pounds, and my life was so limited back then. Now, even though I still have a ways to go, at least I can move around, go for a walk, live like a normal person. The thing is, I snack too much. I still love my crackers and bread, my sweets. I know if I'd just cool it with the snacks, I'd lose more. But they didn't do surgery on my brain, right? My stomach may be smaller, but my head is still the same!"

I couldn't help but love Sharon and her brave, funny, and honest approach to life. But I resolved right then that if God gave me this second chance, I *would* lose all my weight and find a way to keep it off, no matter what it took.

I've been a support group leader for WLS patients at a local hospital for several years, and I've seen hundreds of my fellow surgery recipients make this transformative journey. But like Sharon, many of them never fully achieve their goal. Many have gone back to snacking on foods that are less than optimal, or they don't exercise, or both. And as the statistics on long-term maintenance of this amazing surgery roll in, the emerging picture isn't as encouraging as one would hope. I'll say it again: Many people gain the weight back.

It doesn't have to be that way.

It doesn't even have to be a miserable, awkward struggle to adjust to this new way of life. I've found easy and nurturing ways to take care of myself, and by using these methods I've kept the weight off. I've managed to beat the statistics—and you can too! My life today has moved, as the Overeaters Anonymous literature says, "beyond the food and the emotional havoc into a fuller living experience."

Today I've learned some answers and discovered some tools that really work, not just for the surgery patient, but for anyone who struggles with overeating. They're not the glib answers you'll find on a late-night infomercial, though. Motivational speaker Tony Robbins has said, "Success leaves clues." I will share my clues with you, and I hope you'll be able to find some freedom, as I have. In fact, if you follow some of these clues, I know you will!

How to Get the Most from This Book

Over the years, I've worked with hundreds of clients who were trying to free themselves from a love/hate relationship with a substance or behavior. Whether the addiction is to alcohol, cigarettes, a bad relationship, or food, the process of becoming dependent, hitting bottom, and getting into recovery is remarkably similar. While working in various treatment facilities and private practice, I attended college and obtained state, national, and international credentials as an addictions specialist. And I learned even more from my clients as I supported them through their struggles and successes.

The skills of recovery build on each other, and understanding them is a process, just like learning a foreign language. I will teach you the basics, then we will build on them as you develop the skills needed to take each next step.

Here's what the process is like: Let's say you want to learn to drive a stick-shift car, and I'm your teacher. At the beginning, you know where you want to go; you're just not sure how to get there. Well-meaning people may have given you plenty of advice on how to drive the car, but no one has actually sat down with you and handed you the keys. So you try to take their advice on how to drive, and you get into first gear. You start and stop, start and stall out, start and go five feet, then ten, then a hundred—and then you stall out again!

It's frustrating. Nobody seems to understand why you aren't just driving already. Maybe they think you're stupid, or that there's something wrong with you.

Maybe you think so, too.

I say they're wrong. I say you just haven't had the right teacher, the right information, or the right map!

To get the best results, you'll need to—

o   be willing to try some new tools

o   be motivated enough to use your new tools often

o   consistently practice them until they become habits

o   be willing to stick with the process, remaining patient with yourself through the awkward phase of learning something new

People who know how to drive a stick shift will tell you that they can't remember the exact moment when the learning process went from awkward to easy, from struggle to effortless, but one day they weren't *trying* to drive anymore—they were just driving! The new skill was no longer something outside of themselves; it had become part of them.

For you to get where you want to go—to freedom from food and weight problems—you'll need to try some new tools. If you practice them, they'll become skills. And if you keep on practicing them, one day they'll become more than skills; they'll become a part of you. Then you'll know a real freedom, as well as a sense of peace and pride that no one can take away.

This book is about making changes that will last a lifetime. How you view the process is up to you. If you'd rather go on a quick diet, lose ten pounds before the big day, then go "off the wagon" and gain back twenty, then this book is not for you. Go ahead, go back to the "eat an egg white in the morning and drink cabbage soup at night" plan. But in a year or two, when you've dieted your way up, up, up the scale and are feeling frustrated as hell, I'll still be here.

In a size six.

Here are some of the ways this book differs from the scores of diet books on the shelves:

- I'll present the pros and cons of weight loss surgery, and how to decide if it's right for you.

- I'll show you how to get ready for surgery so your postoperative changes will go smoothly.

- I'll offer helpful post-op tips for one month, three months, six months, one year, and long-term maintenance.

- I'll show you how to get rid of food cravings once and for all.

- I'll show you a way to eat so you won't feel deprived or like you're "missing out."

- You'll learn how to make self-loving changes, instead of using the "drill sergeant" method.

- You'll get so busy doing things you love, you'll forget to eat.

- You'll get clear about what real-life issues the food compulsion or weight problem has been hiding.

o   You'll make friends with your body.

o   You'll get so healthy inside and out that you'll attract great opportunities into your life.

o   One of these opportunities will be to start living your dreams.

Now, doesn't that sound better than the beach club/cabbage soup/protein-till-you-puke diet?

In each chapter you'll find—

o   specific concerns for the WLS patient, including parts of my own story detailing how I learned to deal with the very same issues you may be facing

o   real stories of other WLS patients dealing with their challenges and surmounting them

o   practical suggestions on how you can identify your own problem areas

o   practical assignments to help you find solutions for yourself

These assignments have come straight from my "real world" Overcoming Emotional Eating classes, which are filled with people such as yourself who are struggling with food/weight issues. As you read each chapter, the assignments will help you target which overeating "triggers" are your biggest temptations, and will offer you a variety of tools to deal with them. They will take you on a journey of self-discovery, leading you to your dream destination: a happier, healthier you!

A Bit More about Me

I grew up a fat kid on the California coast, a chubby brunette in a sea of slender blondes. No one else in my immediate family was fat, but they had other problems, including alcoholism, abuse of various sorts, and codependency. Growing up, I learned that the way to deal with uncomfortable feelings was to drink, yell, argue, or, in my case, hide in my bedroom and eat. When I dieted, which was often, I'd lose a little and gain back a lot.

There was a constant war being fought in my head. One side would stand in front of the mirror and say desperately, "How am I gonna lose all this weight?" Then the other side would stand in front of the refrigerator like an eager puppy, saying, "Gee, I wonder what there is to eat?"

Most young adults at my age were putting their energy into marriage and family, but not many guys wanted to marry the fat girl. Or they put their energy into their careers, but not many employers wanted to hire the fat woman. I sacrificed thirty years trying every kind of diet, pill, and gadget to become slender enough to be wanted. If I had the complete answer to why these methods didn't work for me and why WLS did, well, I guess the forty-billion-dollar-a-year diet industry could make me their queen!

By the time I began considering weight loss surgery, I was thirty-eight years old and had been a licensed addictions counselor for over a decade. I had developed a good reputation in both my profession and my personal recovery, because I was able to relate to my clients not just from my university background but "from the trenches"—that is, from a background similar to theirs, as well as from a solid foundation in the twelve steps, which is an excellent framework for personal transformation when dealing with just about any addiction.

After a few years of working in the addiction field, I began writing curriculums used by various treatment programs to rehabilitate their clients, and, hopefully, inspire them into the kind of recovery that lasts. By the time I moved into private practice, I had written and utilized six different twelve-week-long therapeutic curriculums for two treatment centers and one medical program. To date, I've written a total of nine, all of which are still being used today.

After all this spouting off about my accomplishments, you may be wondering, "If she thinks she's so smart, then why couldn't she just stop eating on her own? Why'd she have to have that drastic surgery?"

I have asked myself the same question many, many times. And, as I said, I don't know the whole answer. But I do know some of the pieces....

When I got clean and sober nearly twenty years ago, it wasn't easy, but at least it was *clear*—you get the drugs and alcohol out of your life, period. And while you're at it, you get rid of all the people, places, and things that tempt you to use. Pretty black and white, right? Also, since drugs, alcohol, and cigarettes are generally recognized as health hazards, most people can respect an individual's choice to abstain from them completely.

But how do you do that with food? You have to eat. How do you get *those* people, places, and things out of your life? What if it's your boss or your mother-in-law shoving that tempting little homemade morsel under your nose? Will you offend them by saying no?

All I'm saying is, it ain't easy. If it were, there wouldn't *be* a forty-billion-dollar-a-year diet industry.

It's been several years now since weight loss surgery turned my life around. After the surgery, it took approximately one year for me to lose around 100 pounds. I went from weighing nearly 250 pounds to a current 135 and holding—from a size XXXL to a size six. But it was much more than a physical transformation. Since then, to maintain my weight loss, I've had to learn new ways to deal with my feelings, my actions, other people—in short, everything!

Did I get the great guy? Well, yes and no. You'll have to read my story to find out. Did I find the great career? Did I learn to love myself? Do I feel good every day about what I've learned, and now share with others? Yes and yes and yes!

Whatever you do, even if you don't turn another page, *start by being kind to yourself.* Diets are not kind to the food lover. Society is not kind to the overweight. And many of us have believed the lie that says there is something wrong with us, and we've been hardest of all on ourselves. There is nothing wrong with you—you're fine just the way you are.

Be kind to yourself.

— Michelle Ritchie
Makawao, Hawaii

Weighing the
Pros and Cons of
Weight Loss
Surgery

A guide
to help you make
informed choices

In 2006, over 150,000 weight loss surgeries were performed in the U.S., a tenfold increase in the number of these procedures from 1996. The immediate benefits of the surgery are rapid weight loss, improved vitality and strength, and a return to health and productivity in every aspect of life. We hear miraculous stories of postoperative patients who no longer need their medications because their diabetes, high blood pressure, or high cholesterol goes into remission almost immediately. They feel better, look better, and enjoy far more opportunities in work, love, and personal goals.

It is due to these marvelous changes that so many more people are seeking out WLS (weight loss surgery) today. Just a few years ago, the procedure was virtually unknown; now almost everyone knows someone who has had it done. The *Today* show's Al Roker, *American Idol's* Randy Jackson, Sharon Osborne, even Roseanne Barr have all been candid about their WLS experiences. It's discussed on all the talk shows and throughout the media. There are even TV commercials promoting the surgery by showing true "before and after" stories.

But along with these happy results, there is another side to the story that has been underreported. Often patients who undergo WLS aren't given enough support, education, and guidance to make it a long-term success. Yes, they lose weight initially—but often gain it back. Yes, some health conditions improve dramatically as the weight comes off; however, WLS can also exacerbate or even cause certain health problems.

Whether the type of surgery is gastric bypass, lap-band, or some other variation on what used to be called "stomach stapling," in essence they all drastically reduce the size of the stomach, from a capacity of approximately four or five cups of food at a time to a capacity of one ounce. That's one ounce, folks. Smaller than a golf ball, and only slightly bigger than a grape. Simply put, if the patient is used to eating larger than normal amounts of food, and if they are used to eating for comfort or to deal with frustration or worry, then once the surgery is over they're in for a shock. Food—their solace, their lover, their buffer, their reward—is gone. It's just not possible to use that coping method anymore, unless they want to end up in the emergency room! And, unless they learn new skills, after the first year when their new "pouch" stretches and their food cravings return, many WLS post-ops put the pounds back on.

But this doesn't have to be the case. Weight loss surgery can be—and remain—a success!

This book is written to help two groups of people. First, it's for those dealing with WLS, to inform and support them before, during, and after the process. We will look at preoperative considerations, what the surgery itself is like, the process of losing over a hundred pounds, and, finally, how to maintain a healthy body and mindset once the weight is off.

The book is also for anyone who wants freedom from food obsession and excess weight—anyone who has suffered from compulsive overeating and body image issues. The methods outlined in this book will work for both groups by providing practical solutions for weight loss *and* maintenance.

Right about here you may be wondering, "But why do I have do worry about 'methods' if I'm going to have WLS? Won't the surgery just do the job for me?"

So, which do you want first, the good news or the bad news?

First, the good news. The methods in this book, although they do include some suggestions for a food plan, are *not* another diet. In fact, I strongly encourage you to never diet again. Here is your first freedom —freedom from the tyranny of the diet mentality!

Now for the other news. *Weight loss surgery is not a miracle cure.* Many people have gone through this very serious procedure without making any other changes in their lives—and they soon gained all their weight back, or never lost much to begin with.

How could that be possible with such a tiny stomach, you ask? Well, first of all, the stomach doesn't *stay* so small. By eighteen to twenty-four months after surgery it has typically stretched out enough to accommodate a small, relatively normal-sized meal. Also, the cravings to eat sugary or starchy foods, which often disappear initially, usually return after about six to twelve months post-op, and if you give in to them you can certainly eat small amounts of ice cream and cookies and whatever else you want—and end up gaining weight just like anyone else!

The surgery is just a tool. It can jump-start the weight loss process by making it impossible to eat large amounts of food during the first eighteen months after surgery—but that's all. It is *crucial* to use the "window of opportunity" provided by the first year post-op to make the emotional, mental, and lifestyle changes that will maintain a healthy body over the long term. Otherwise, you could have the surgery, deal with the year-long healing process afterward, and go through all of it for nothing.

In addition to the small size of the stomach, when the method used is gastric bypass, the surgeon will remove three to six feet of intestines, reducing the body's ability to metabolize and retain fats and sugars and thus assisting in weight loss. This is a double-edged sword, however, because the lack of intestines also means that forever afterward, the postoperative WLS patient must take daily vitamin supplements and be very careful about getting all of their nutritional needs met.

Furthermore, the lack of intestines doesn't allow for sugars or fats to be processed in the usual manner; thus, the post-op WLS patient can experience an unpleasant physical reaction to sugary or fatty foods called "dumping," which provides a kind of negative support. Dumping makes you feel so bad (with reactions like instant diarrhea, flatulence, and sweating) that you don't want to keep doing it. For some people, this negative feedback helps them stay away from those kinds of foods.

Like many others, I was a "poster child" after the surgery, with no major complications, no dumping, nothing but positive results. If I wanted to, I could eat small bowls of Häagen-Dazs all day long with no negative reactions—except of course, the weight gain! I'll say it again:

The surgery is only a tool, and you'll need to make other important life-style changes if you want to get healthy and stay that way.

Getting Ready for Change
◎

A number of studies have been conducted over the past few years concerning how and why people change. Psychologists and scientific researchers have interviewed hundreds of subjects who were trying to quit smoking, get off alcohol or other drugs, or change other undesirable habits. What they found, as they followed these people through their process of change, was a series of steps that each person typically goes through in order to be successful. The first three steps are sometimes called precontemplation, contemplation, and preparation. I call them "getting ready for change."

Why would "getting ready" for a change be important? Don't we simply get fed up and then "just do it," like the Nike commercials say? Well, I tried dieting that way many, many times—tried and failed. I'd get sick of how I looked, sick of how I felt, and go on a diet. There was the cabbage soup diet, the macrobiotic diet, the Hollywood diet, the low-fat/low-sugar/low-carb diet. There was Dr. Atkins, Dr. Pritikin, and Dr. Phil. There was the one where you only drink apple juice for a week, then down a cup of olive oil (yuck!). There was the one where you only drink lemon water with cayenne pepper and a dash of honey for as many days as you can stand it. Crazy or not, if it promised quick results, I'd go for it—because, of course, I wanted to hurry up and get back to eating once the weight was off.

Problem was, none of these plans was sustainable over the long haul. They all involved some kind of deprivation, and as we all know the more we tell ourselves we *can't* have something, the more we want it—until we give in, go on a binge, and eat everything in sight. Then, like an alcoholic's "morning after," we feel sick, guilty, and swear off forever—until the next time.

Trying to change without any preparation is like planting a seedling without tilling the soil. If I just cram its fragile roots into the hard ground, how long is it likely to live? Not long, just like my shaky motivation. But if I do the groundwork, add some fertilizer, and nurture its development, then the seedling, like any changes I want to make, stands a much better chance of growing strong.

Often a turning point occurs because there has been a crisis in our lives. Maybe a doctor has told us we're on the verge of diabetes or heart trouble; maybe a loved one has confronted us about our weight; maybe none of our clothes fit anymore and we don't want to buy bigger ones. This point of emotional or physical crisis has caused many people to consider having weight loss surgery.

Whatever the wake-up call is for you, it's important to really look at it, and to feel the emotions that go with it—feel the sadness, frustration, even despair.

Then, take it a step further and ask yourself, "If I keep going the way I'm going now, where will my life be in a year? In five years?"

Many of us call this point of critical self-awareness "hitting bottom." It means we've gone as far down as we can go, and we realize we *must* make a change. Because if we don't, we stand to lose something precious.

In my case, my failing marriage served as a wake-up call. . . .

Hitting Bottom

◉

I'd been so happy to marry Eric. It wasn't like I was the fat girl who settled for some loser, no indeed. He was sweet, handsome, kind, and loving, everything a girl could want. He saw me as beautiful, despite the fact that I weighed in at two hundred pounds on our wedding day. We entered into our marriage with so much love, so much in common, happy and hopeful about our future together.

Sadly, the insecurities we'd both tried to suppress when we were engaged came out with a vengeance once we were married. My fears were mostly about being the fat girl married to the good-looking guy, so whenever I saw women staring at Eric, I'd get upset and act jealous. Then he'd get upset at me, thinking I didn't trust him! Round and round we went, spiraling downward, our happy moments overshadowed by destructive bickering over the next few years, until we were both too hurt and too weary to keep going.

In my sad confusion, looking for answers, I spent several hours one night reviewing my journals from the previous years, where I'd written just about everything about my life.

Reading my diaries left me with some startling insights. I had never before realized what a big role my problems with food and weight had played in our relationship. I believed that because I was fat, I must be worthless, so how could he really love me? And from that way of thinking grew the rest of my problems, all sorts of jealousies and insecurities, fears that he'd find someone better—meaning thinner.

Throughout my marital challenges, to cover my anxiety, I ate. The bigger I got, the more my insecurities flared up—and the roller-coaster ride would begin again. I was stuck in the vicious cycle of hurting and hating myself around food. The real irony was that Eric didn't even care about my weight. It would go up, then down; he rarely even noticed. It wasn't an issue for him like it was for me. But I managed to make it "our" problem anyway!

After reading my journals, I came to the conclusion that I had to *do something*—not just about my weight, but about the fearful, wounded part of me that kept sabotaging every happy thing in my life. So I prayed and asked for direction from Spirit. Just two days later, I saw my first TV show on weight loss surgery.

Coincidence? I think not.

It took ten or eleven months from the time I began to research weight loss surgery before I actually underwent the procedure. Once I learned that my HMO had a whole department dealing with WLS and offered a support group for it, I was convinced. Because I knew that weight loss alone wouldn't be a magical cure, I also began to use therapy, meditation, and exercise to help me deal with the changes that were to come. With a little luck and a lot of hard work, maybe I could save my marriage, I thought.

And if not, at least I could save myself.

So that was what it took for me to "hit bottom." My health was poor in every area, physically, mentally, and emotionally. My marriage was failing, and I could clearly see the connection between the problems in my life and my food/weight issues.

Even though I was still getting some comfort from food—at least in the short term—the more I looked at the bigger picture, the more I realized that I did *not* want to spend the rest of my life in this depressing daily battle, one that I lost more often than not!

If you're reading this book, chances are you, too, have already gone through many painful moments as a result of your eating habits and/or weight. If you are considering weight loss surgery, it's important to assess the pros and cons of this decision and to be clear that you believe it is a necessity for your overall health. Once you've completed this chapter's assignments, you will have all the information you need to make your decision.

Is Weight Loss Surgery Right for You?

The first step is to become clear about where you stand, about whether or not WLS surgery is what you really want. This procedure has proved to be a lifesaving intervention for many, many people—yet it is not without risk. Approximately one in two hundred die from it, and many more endure at least some complications. The complications range from minor, temporary concerns, like nausea or vomiting in the first few months after surgery, to varying degrees of malnutrition and the problems that go with it.

Many chronically obese people are already dealing with serious health concerns, however, and the idea of going through a few minor hurdles as the weight comes off doesn't faze them. "I'd been dealing with asthma, diabetes, and joint pain on a daily basis for years, and it was just getting worse," one patient said. "When I looked over the rate of complications resulting from this surgery and compared it to the problems I was already having because of my weight, it seemed like an acceptable risk."

For many of us, the health problems we already had were getting worse over the months and years as we tried to "diet" and then gave up, overate, and stalled in our weight loss when the diets didn't do enough.

Why was our health getting worse? Because any disease process is progressive; it doesn't stay the same. Because the kind of vigorous exercise that could help to relieve these problems was often impossible, due to our health already being so poor that we could hardly walk or breathe.

Here is one of the biggest hurdles to jump over in your decision-making process about WLS. Ask yourself: Do I still feel that I can lose this weight on my own? Or is it time to accept the evidence—that I've tried and failed with the dieting method so many times, and I haven't had any lasting success. Do I want to sacrifice any more years of my life waiting for the next miracle diet to do the trick?

It's normal to feel apprehensive when approaching any big decision, and more so when there are significant risks involved. But all of life is a series of choices and calculated risks, some of which are worth taking, in the hopes of creating a better life.

Many clinics that perform weight loss surgery have a series of tests that the WLS candidate must pass, including a psychological exam, a physical exam, and a pre-op therapy program. Many offer support groups and counseling both before and after surgery. I urge you to take advantage of these tools to help you make your decision.

◎   ◎   ◎

ASSIGNMENT: A Self-Assessment—Getting Ready for Change

This assignment takes a little time, but I strongly encourage you to do it. It's worth a half hour or an hour of your time to be clear and compassionate in your understanding of yourself and to become rock solid in your motivation if you decide to follow through with WLS.

To do this exercise, you'll need—

○ a blank journal and a pen (you'll use this journal often as you go through the helpful assignments in the rest of the book)

○ a glass of water or herb tea (because answering these questions may bring up feelings and make you want to eat, so have the water or tea instead)

○ some quiet space and time away from distractions (thirty to sixty minutes, possibly over two sessions)

○ willingness to be open-minded and honest with yourself

○ willingness to acknowledge and stay with your feelings as they arise and evolve

Please answer the following questions in detail:

1. What kinds of crazy behavior have you engaged in that involved eating (for example, eating food you'd bought for others or food that was harmful to your health)?

2. Did you ever hide food, sneak food, or promise to save some for later but then end up eating it all?

3. Did you ever keep eating past the point of fullness?

4. Did you try to hide these behaviors from others?

5. Did some of these things happen repeatedly, even though you promised yourself you'd stop?

6. How did you feel about yourself when you engaged in any of the above behaviors with food? Did you ever feel ashamed, inferior, weak, screwed up, or even worthless? Did you try to hide these feelings from others?

7. Did you have a frequent underlying feeling of depression, low self-esteem, or hopelessness? Give at least two examples of

the underlying feelings you've experienced and how they have affected your life.

8. Did you occasionally tell yourself, "I've got to change this," but then go right back to overeating?

9. How many diets, diet pills, or other weight loss schemes have you tried? List them all. Then ask yourself as honestly as possible, "Have I been able to lose weight and *maintain* the loss through these methods?"

10. What were the triggers that tempted you back into overeating?

11. As well as you can remember, list your weight ranges by decade and consider how they have changed over your lifetime. For example, "In my teens I weighed 150–175 pounds, in my twenties I averaged 160–200 pounds, and in my thirties I was 170–250 pounds. In each decade my weight always went up and down as I yo-yo dieted my way up the scale." Ask yourself again, "Have I gotten the long-term results I want through dieting?"

12. How did your overeating affect you physically? List at least five ways, either health concerns you have had or physical things you couldn't or wouldn't do because of food and weight problems (e.g., wear shorts, go to the beach, go dancing, go hiking, etc.).

13. How have weight/food issues affected your relationships with those you love? List three ways.

14. Did you ever isolate yourself from others because of your food obsession or weight?

15. Have you ever tried to be extra giving or extra friendly to others to "make up" for the fact that you were big? If yes, how did this make you feel?

16. How have food/weight issues affected your social life in general? List three ways.

17. How have food/weight issues affected your life at school or work? List three ways.

18. Do you feel that these issues have held you back from becoming all you could be in your career or other goals? How?

19. How have your problems with food/weight affected your spiritual life (i.e., your beliefs about life and about yourself, and your relationship with Spirit/God/the world)?

20. What other ways have food/weight issues impacted your life? For example, how much money, how much time, and how many opportunities have you lost due to these problems? List at least one example for each area.

If you've done a sincere job answering the above questions, you may be experiencing some uncomfortable feelings. Sorry. But it's important to really see and feel and realize all that you are missing or stand to lose by continuing the same old patterns related to food and weight. It is a paradox in recovery that sometimes our most hurtful memories can become our closest friends, because keeping them fresh reminds us of the important reasons why we *don't* want to go back down that old, familiar road.

At this point, you may feel tempted to berate yourself, feel horrible about yourself, or wonder why the hell you are like this and if it will ever get any better. If so, I want to really encourage you to do two things:

1. Allow any feelings you have to come out. Cry if you need to. Tell that self-critical inner voice to take a hike—just get rid of it. What good did it ever do anyway?

2. Remind yourself that your old eating behaviors were really coping skills—not the best ones, maybe, but coping skills nonetheless. They helped you get through some rough times with a little nurturing, and we all need that, don't we? So rather than beating yourself up over the past, acknowledge that, hey, you've made it this far! You're still here. You survived, and there were times when those old coping skills helped you do it.

And now, like a snake shedding its skin, you can—gently and at your own pace—let go of them in favor of a truer nourishment.

Like what?

I'll show you as we go along.

Practical Considerations

◎

I don't need to tell you that choosing WLS is a major, life-changing, very big decision, right? Because of this, I highly recommend that you do as much research as you can so you will feel that you are fully informed about the pros and cons of the procedure, including potential risks as well as benefits. The following websites are excellent resources to assist you in learning everything you can about WLS:

www.obesityhelp.com

www.wlscenter.com

www.onpointhealth.com

www.nlm.nih.gov (this is Medline Plus, operated by the federal government)

www.weightlosssurgeryoptions.com

(Each of these is listed again in the Resources section, located at the back of the book.)

The above sites provide the most neutral information I could find. There are plenty of other websites that discuss WLS, but most of them are run by clinics, doctors, or others who have something to gain by influencing your decision. Please bear in mind that any site that is run for profit may emphasize only the positive side of the story!

Take the time to explore these sites and any others that interest you. Once you've done so, you'll be ready for the next steps in the process.

If your research, in conjunction with completing the first assignment, has helped you conclude that WLS is right for you, the next step is to approach your medical insurance company. The most common prerequisites for weight loss surgery include the following:

- A history of chronic obesity.

- A history of failed methods of losing weight, including diets, exercise, and/or medications such as Meridia or Xenical. You'll need to document these in detail.

- A body mass index (BMI) of forty or above. A BMI of thirty-five or above may qualify you if you also have significant weight-related health problems, such as diabetes, asthma, sleep apnea, heart problems, high blood pressure, or a family history of these concerns. (These are called "comorbidities" in medical terminology.) To determine your BMI, just log on to www.obesityhelp.com and follow the directions. The site will calculate your BMI for you, along with offering lots of other helpful information on WLS.

If you meet these qualifications, many health insurance providers will pay for your weight loss surgery with a minimal copayment on your part. In fact, more and more HMOs are opting to pay for the surgery with an eye toward the future; their reasoning is that if an obese person loses most of their excess weight via surgery, then they'll cost their insurance provider less over the long haul since they'll probably avoid further medical expenses triggered by other chronic conditions.

What Fat People Can't Do

Not everything about WLS has to be deep, serious, and profound. One of my greatest tools throughout this process has been to find some humor in my situation wherever I can. At the WLS support groups that I facilitate, sometimes we end up roaring with laughter over the strangest things! In that spirit, I've included a serious (but not too serious) list for you to consider.

We all live by a lot of unspoken cultural rules. They're not laws; you can't get arrested for breaking them—but if you go against the social code you'll feel the burn almost immediately. Sure, some people love to rebel, and they'll push the envelope just for shock value, but the average Joe feels a certain safety in following the herd. And that goes for most of us.

Maybe you think I'm exaggerating. Or maybe you think you're better than that, that your strength of character rises above that of the masses, and that society's displeasure couldn't faze you. I'd like to believe that about myself, but having lived most of my life as a fat woman, I know better.

If you think you're immune to public opinion, try this experiment. Go downtown on any weekday wearing only a pair of boxer shorts. If you're a woman, go wearing boxer shorts and a plain white bra. Now, you're not exactly indecent or naked in this outfit—you're wearing just as much clothing as you would at the beach, right? Here in Hawaii, plenty of teenage girls wear surf shorts and little sport tops no bigger than a bra, or a bikini top with shorts. On the weekends you can see herds of high school girls roaming the malls in this uniform and no one thinks anything of it. What's the big difference between swim clothes and underclothes?

So, would you try my experiment?

I didn't think so.

And if you wouldn't, then have some compassion for the rough road that an obese person travels through a hostile society. Have some compassion for yourself.

Here are some of our unspoken rules:

o   Don't go to the beach.

o   Don't wear shorts.

o   Don't go out to dance at a club.

o   Don't assume thin people want to have anything to do with you.

o Don't wear white; it makes you look bigger.

o Don't wear anything sleeveless.

o Don't apply for most jobs.

o Don't make eye contact.

o Don't eat in front of anybody, or if you must, eat salad.

o Don't take up too much space.

o Don't do anything that might make your fat jiggle in public.

o Don't make love with the lights on.

o Don't expect to make love at all.

o Don't let anyone see your body.

o Don't try new things socially.

o Don't stand up for yourself; just swallow it.

o Don't expect much real happiness.

o Don't expect fair treatment or real respect.

o Don't go grocery shopping at rush hour.

o In fact, just don't go grocery shopping.

o Don't go clothes shopping.

o Don't walk down a street when you can drive; driving is better because no one can really see you.

o Do extra well at work; take on double the load.

o Do take on everybody's burdens so you'll be needed even though you're fat.

o Do be overly grateful when anyone is nice to you.

o Do be extra friendly to make up for being fat.

o Do make jokes about your fat before anyone else does.

o Do wear black or dark colors, nothing bright.

o Do wear dark, loose clothes that cover your body, look at the ground as you walk, try to stay out of people's way, and say "sorry" and "excuse me" a lot.

It's a heck of a way to live!

ASSIGNMENT: How I'm Limited Because of My Weight

In the above list you can see some of the limitations I used to put on myself because of my weight. Most of mine had to do with being judged by other people—which you surely understand if you have walked through our society in an overweight body for any length of time. But at 250 pounds I was still able to move around, fit into most chairs, even squeeze myself (barely) into an airplane seat!

For those of us who have moved beyond the XXL range and can't "fit in"—literally—to many of the chairs, booths, opportunities, and ideals that our society offers, how much more are we limited? I know many beautiful souls whose weight has limited them to a very small life in a very small space—a chair in their house, a corner of the couch, or a bed. We deserve so much more than this. We deserve all that life has to offer!

So whether your "range of motion" is limited by the confines of your body, the confines of your mind and heart, or the confines of our society, take some time now to write down all the things you can't or won't do because of your weight. Complete the following sentences in writing. Maybe you have more than one response to some of them. Write down all responses that come to mind.

1. Because of my body's physical limits right now, I can't...
2. If my body were fit and healthy, I would like to...
3. Because of the way my body looks, I don't...
4. If my body looked great, I would...
5. If I felt better about myself, I'd like to try...
6. If I had wonderful self-confidence, I would...
7. The dreams I've put on hold because of my weight are...
8. If I keep going the way I have been with my food and body issues, in five years my life will be...
9. If I make these healthy changes with my food and body issues, in five years my life could be...

Really looking at your answers to these questions can give you a clearer picture of what you've given up or what you may further lose if you don't take a stand for your health. Once you've completed the assignments in this chapter, you will, as I promised, have a pretty good idea of where you want to go from here. And once you've decided where you want to go, we'll talk about how you can get there!

◎ Sue's Story

Sue is a thirty-seven-year-old mother of three who gained seventy-five pounds and became prediabetic while juggling family and her own business. I met her in my OEE (Overcoming Emotional Eating) class, where she came seeking answers to the issues of her weight, her daily fatigue, and her attempts to keep up with the pace of her work and kids.

"I kept going back and forth about whether or not to have the surgery," she said, "because my general health wasn't that bad. I knew that the overall risks weren't too severe, but still, they said one patient in two hundred die as a result of it, and I had my kids to think about. I kept on trying to diet, and over the next year or so I'd go up and down maybe five or ten pounds, but the major change I was hoping to make just didn't happen. So I decided to go for it.

"I was scared, but I did meet a lot of other post-ops at our local WLS support group who reassured me. Some of them even visited me in the hospital after surgery. It's been about seven months now since I had my surgery. I've lost most of the extra weight, and I'm no longer prediabetic. I can't say it's been easy, but it's been worth it, and I'm looking forward to even better health in the future."

chapter
two

Preparing
the
Path to Freedom

*Laying the
foundations*

28

About eighteen months after WLS, I underwent reconstructive surgery to remove some of the skin that was left over from my loss of more than a hundred pounds. The doctor gave me a long list of foods to avoid as I prepared for surgery, including coffee. Now, I've been the Coffee Queen since I was eighteen years old, to the point where my friends tease me about my love affair with it. I enjoy the ritual of going to the coffeehouse, ordering my special coffee drink, and hanging out with friends there. I never *really* overdo it, I tell myself. Besides, after giving up booze, drugs, cigarettes, sugar, wheat products, dangerous men, and swearing, I was very self-righteous about the whole thing. "It's my last vice," I'd tell people. "So just leave me alone about it. I've got to have *something*, don't I?"

But now I was facing expensive elective surgery, and the doctor was very clear about it.

Give up coffee? Geez.

I decided to apply everything I'd learned from all the other bad habits I'd given up, to see if I could make it a smooth transition. Here is what I did:

o   I made a plan, which I wrote on the calendar, to slowly wean myself off coffee over a three-week period.

o   I told everyone close to me what I was doing so I couldn't sneak it in when I was around them.

o   I slowly replaced regular coffee with decaf, using a little more decaf and a little less regular coffee each day.

o   I treated myself to the fanciest gourmet decaf I could buy. It actually tasted better than the real thing!

o   I cut out other caffeine products, replacing them with caffeine-free alternatives.

o   To combat the cravings and fatigue that arose from getting off caffeine, I took the amino acids L-glutamine and DL-phenylalanine daily, along with my vitamins, for two months (more on amino acid supplements later).

o As I progressed to being caffeine-free, I allowed myself to feel proud of my accomplishment, and I shared my progress with my friends.

After twenty-two years as a caffeine addict, letting go of it was so smooth that I barely even noticed it.

Why am I sharing this story about coffee with you when I know you are facing a much bigger lifestyle shift with WLS and food? Because it illustrates how to utilize some of the same tools that are very effective when changing your eating habits. Make no mistake, even after you undergo surgery, it is still an absolute necessity to use whatever tools you have available to jump-start a lifestyle change regarding food. Yes, the surgery will do the work for you—for the first twelve to eighteen months. During that time, most people report very little hunger and few cravings. They eat only enough to nourish their bodies, and they take care to avoid stretching their newly small stomach "pouch."

But, as is the case with many things, familiarity breeds carelessness, and, in time, the cravings come back, the new pouch stretches, and it becomes possible once again to eat your way back up to your starting weight. Sound familiar? That is why the next stage of change, from preparation into action, is so critical. It calls for you to get yourself, your loved ones, and your kitchen ready for the healthy shift you are about to make.

Realize, too, that as much as you may have been looking forward to having the surgery, it often seems like a fantasy cure—that is, until you are given a surgery date and come face to face with some feelings you didn't expect! This chapter will help you make a concrete plan of action for the first stages of change that are involved in preparing for weight loss surgery. If you've already had the surgery, the chapter will help you develop a plan for beginning the lifestyle changes that will make it a lasting success.

Last of the Last Suppers

I first approached my insurance provider about WLS in July of 2001. By the time I was finally approved for the procedure it was February 2002, eight months later. So I'd been in a mindset that said "I'm about to have this life-changing surgery any minute now" for quite some time, and I had even gotten used to the idea. My slightly less obese friends said they envied me. "I wish I could do it too," they'd say with longing, as if it were just another diet pill or cellulite cream or exercise machine they could try and then abandon, as we had all done so many times before.

By that time, however, I knew better. The work the medical team did during the waiting period was profound. They didn't just tell me what to expect after surgery; they showed me. I attended several support group meetings of patients who'd had the surgery before me, a group that numbered close to one hundred people. It was from these brave souls that I learned the most. Some breezed through the procedure and dropped a hundred pounds or more in the following months with nary a catch.

But not all. Some of them had a very difficult time during the first few months post-op. The least of what they endured was bouts of nausea and vomiting in the process of learning what their new "baby stomachs" could handle. Some foods would be fine one day but would make them throw up the next. The group members also were very fond of showing off their scars. I saw tummy tucks and arm skin reductions. I also saw open wounds that hadn't healed even months after surgery. I heard about patients too sick to attend the meetings, some still in the hospital fighting for their lives after surgery-related complications. These weren't just stories on the Internet anymore; they were real people right in front of me. Seeing an open wound on someone's midriff when they lifted up their shirt—whew. It was a hell of a reality check.

But that is exactly what it should be. I mean, consider: They cut your stomach apart, staple the parts shut, then cut out three to six feet of your intestines. This is some serious tinkering with your system, and if you're not ready to deal with *all* the possible realities—not just pretty pictures of those who lost weight—you shouldn't get into the game in the first place.

Funny thing, though. Even the lady with the scary open wound was smiling and laughing as she talked to her post-op buddies. Even those who told gory stories of their ordeal showed up at the support meetings as the confident, happy people they had become. And almost all said, "I'd do it again in a heartbeat. It changed my life—I *have* a life today. I feel so proud of myself, so good about who I am becoming." One woman had become a marathon runner. Another opened a business doing something she'd always dreamed about but had lacked the confidence to try. They used words like "released" and "freed" and "grateful." I remember the looks on their faces: sincere, down to earth, smiling—and profoundly relieved.

On the last night that I was allowed to eat before surgery, I had the Last Supper of all Last Suppers. (I got that term from an *Oprah* show on dieting in which she joked with the audience, "How many Last Suppers before the big diet have you all had? I know I've had plenty!") After that, I would have to throw away all the pastries, pastas, cheeses, chips, brownies—you name it—because I had to go on clear liquids to prepare for surgery. I thought I would go out with friends and make a big deal of my last "food fest," but I couldn't. I was ashamed, because I knew that I had hurt myself with this "food-disease" to the point where I saw the surgery as my only hope. This made it kind of hard to go out and eat with everybody, pretending that it was all just a big piggie celebration. It would have felt kind of crazy, like I was mainlining heroin in front of a crowd. I couldn't do it. I ended up eating at home, in isolation once again. It all felt so very familiar. How many times in the past had I thrown food away after Last Suppers? How many times had I gone out and bought more the next day? How many hundreds of dollars and how many years of my life had I thrown away in the process? And yet people actually still question if this is really an addiction? Please.

As the preparation process for weight loss surgery has improved over the years, most WLS programs now realize that many of their preoperative patients tend go on a "last supper" binge like I did, further endangering their health. Nowadays, preoperative guidelines are much stricter about diet and weight gain prior to WLS, and I fully support these changes.

◎ Bill's Story

I salute the brave men who have stuck it out in my classes—because usually they are far outnumbered by the women! But society's pressure to look good at any price has definitely become a co-ed issue, and men feel this stress, too. Although men and women do have special concerns specific to their gender, there are also many similarities in their experience—such as eating to overcome negative feelings, eating due to stress, trying to be fit enough for a good job or relationship, and struggling to feel good about themselves.

My client Bill, a dynamic fifty-eight-year-old financial analyst, had lived the full spectrum of body types over the last forty years—from being a college football player, to becoming alarmingly thin during his workaholic thirties and forties, to becoming overweight after a car accident caused a spinal injury at age fifty. As a result of his injury, Bill had cut back on all of his athletic activities, and, frustrated with his forced idleness, he came to my OEE class.

"I've always been the kind of man to 'go forth and conquer' whatever I wanted in my life," Bill shared with the group. "So when it came to a situation where all I could do was be gentle, go slow, and take it easy on my back so it wouldn't get worse, well, let's just say that taking it easy was not exactly my comfort zone. I found myself eating due to frustration, and along with the inactivity, my weight started to climb. Michelle's class helped me to take a broader view of what was missing in my life. I came to realize that

(cont'd.)

everybody needs nurturing, even us men! And I realized that I had gone from getting my enjoyment from sports to finding a pseudo-satisfaction in food and snacking in front of ESPN.

"Probably my biggest 'aha' experience from the class was trying to answer Michelle's question, 'What does it mean to really love and nurture yourself?' I realized that without ever thinking about it, I'd bought into the TV and media answer: eating yummy fast food as a form of nurturing.

"But when I went deeper in my thinking and feeling about what it **really** means to love yourself, I found myself remembering my football days, and how good it felt to be fit and strong instead of tired and sluggish from eating crummy fake burgers and fries!

"Now, even though I'm certainly not twenty anymore and have injuries that won't allow me to go back to the level of fitness I'd like, that doesn't mean I have to give up and make things worse with junk foods that, far from being nurturing, are actually abusive to my body. There are still lots of other ways I can become healthier and feel better in the body I have. What it means to love and nurture myself has become a more important question, with a more mature answer. It means to take good care of myself rather than going for a quick fix that makes me feel worse later on."

So, dear reader, consider: What does it mean to you to truly love and nurture yourself?

Beginning to Change: Nurturing Your Body

One of the primary reasons why most diets fail is because they don't do anything to stop food cravings. Whether you begin the lifestyle shift outlined in this book before having weight loss surgery or after (I suggest doing it before), any food plan you try to follow will be a lot easier if you can manage to reduce or eliminate cravings. As I've said, WLS may handle your food cravings for the first few months, but unfortu-nately, *they come back.*

Cravings—for sweets, for salty or fried foods, for comfort, for re-laxation, for nurturing—are the termites that undermine even our strongest determination and can eventually set us off on a binge. We try heroically to keep our mind on our weight loss goal while the rest of our system is calling out for that old familiar fix. Whether our cravings are for chocolate, french fries, ice cream, or whatever, they can steadily eat away at your resolve until you give in.

So the first and most important step is to support and nourish your physical body in such a way that it doesn't kick and scream for Häagen-Dazs or Doritos while you're trying your best to follow a food plan.

As you look for a nutrition plan that will work for you, bear in mind that there are several principles that can make the transition much easier—like my strategy of switching from real coffee to decaf. Here are some of them:

Let go of dieting. Diets don't work. Stop dieting forever, because di-eting deprivation triggers overeating. Instead, focus on making small, consistent steps that will create a lasting lifestyle change.

Let go of the black-and-white thinking that goes along with dieting. Thoughts like, "When I'm 'on the wagon' I have to be perfect, deprive myself, never have foods I like. When I'm 'off the wagon' I can really go for it, have as much as I want of whatever I want." Neither of these methods can be maintained for very long, and often we ricochet back and forth between the two.

Use a multidimensional approach. Nourish the body, nurture the heart and spirit, retrain and refocus the mind. It's important to address all these areas, as well as our social interactions and relationships, in or-der to be successful over the long term. I will provide suggestions and tools for how to do this in upcoming chapters.

Let go of trigger foods. These are the foods that call your name late at night and whisper to you when you're trying to get through the day, the ones you miss most when you diet and the first thing you eat when you go off a diet. I can't give you an exact formula for your own trigger foods, but many people identify sweets, starchy foods, chocolate, fast foods, and fried foods. After many years of trial and error, I try to practice zero tolerance with my trigger foods. If I don't eat it, I won't crave it. If I have even a little, I will want more, and even today, my so-called willpower isn't always up to the task of fighting those cravings. So I don't eat wheat, sugar, fast foods, or junk foods.

Now, you may not need to be as strict as I am on this issue. You can always experiment a bit to see if you can have a small portion of your trigger foods without setting off monster cravings or a binge, or if, like me, you find it's just simpler to abstain entirely. This strategy can be made easier if you also follow the next one.

Find a substitute for your trigger foods so you don't feel deprived. This is one of the most important strategies for any kind of change—finding something healthy to replace the negative thing you are letting go of. In my house I keep sugar-free hot cocoa, sugar-free chocolate and candy (Russell Stover's brand), fat-free chips, and fat-free popcorn. Some part of me feels better just knowing that these little "treats" are there, that I can have them if I want them. Because I give myself permission to do that, and *because they don't contain my trigger foods,* I don't overeat them. I eat maybe one piece of sugar-free candy or a handful of fat-free chips every two or three days. I also try to be careful not to eat mindlessly when I really need to be dealing head-on with some feeling or situation. No doubt a health-food purist would object to using these substitutes and would suggest fruits instead. That's great if fruit does it for you; it certainly is a healthier choice. But for me, having those pseudo-treats in the house helps me play a little Jedi mind trick on myself. I tell myself, "You are not being deprived; you can still have treats," even though I rarely eat them. And for this lifetime foodaholic, it works. However, if at some point I did start to overeat these foods, I'd get them out of the house. Which brings me to our next strategy...

Make a temptation-free space in your home and wherever else you can. Ideally, remove all trigger foods from your home so you won't even be tempted. Ask the people you live with if they'll work with you on this issue. Even if they aren't willing to get those foods completely out of the house, they may be willing to put them in a place where you don't have to look at them every time you open the fridge or kitchen cabinet.

At work, many of us have to endure a daily array of pastries, candies, and cookies in the employee lounge or kitchen. At my old job, even if I avoided the kitchen, people would come around to my desk and offer me "treats" filled with sugar and starch. Of course, they didn't realize what they were doing—they were just being nice. I managed to find friendly ways to thank them for the offer but to say, "No, I don't do sugar," and, "No, it's not a diet," and "Thanks anyway but, no, I can't have just one." Then I'd find a casual, joking way to say, "And by the way, keep your temptations to yourself, okay?" It's often hard to ask for this kind of support; we feel awkward or foolish, or like we don't have the right to "bother" those we live or work with. However, if you are serious about making this change, you have to be willing to go the extra mile to help yourself, and sometimes this involves asking for support from others. I have found that if we ask in a courteous manner, people are usually willing to work with us.

Use vitamins and amino acid therapy to get you over the withdrawal period. Make no mistake, trigger foods have their own withdrawal syndrome, just like letting go of a drug. You may experience mood swings, feel irritable, and battle cravings for the foods you are letting go of. In Appendix A, I give specific formulas for using amino acid therapy to facilitate a smooth withdrawal period from a variety of foods. Regarding vitamins, if you are a postoperative gastric bypass patient, you will need to take at least double the daily RDA of vitamins and minerals for the rest of your life. This is because the same intestinal bypass procedure that reduces your ability to absorb fats also reduces your ability to metabolize other nutrients, and it's important to make sure you don't become malnourished or ill from any vitamin or mineral deficiencies. Taking extra iron, calcium citrate, and B vitamins, especially sublingual B-12, is necessary. Discuss this with your doctor and make sure you clearly understand the dosages you will be expected to take, and for how long.

Eat at least 60 grams of protein daily, eat lots of fresh vegetables and fruits, and drink plenty of water. Consume these foods in five to six small meals per day, or, if you prefer, in three meals and two snacks. This is a formula that doctors have been recommending for decades to hypoglycemic and diabetic patients. It also works very well for those of us who tend to crave carbs, carbs, and more carbs. It helps to regulate blood sugar, stabilize moods, and eliminate cravings. A disclaimer here, though: If your kidneys, cholesterol levels, or any other aspect of your health is not up to par, please work with your doctor to tailor your nutritional plan to meet your specific needs.

ASSIGNMENT: My Nurturing Food Plan

With the food plan we're about to develop, you won't be hungry, and you'll feel full, satisfied, and content. You'll get to have treats, and your overall energy level and mood will be consistent throughout the day. You'll have friends, family, and would-be scoffers leaning over your shoulder to see what's in *your* lunch, saying, "Hey, that looks good—did you make that? I wish I could get it together enough to do that." You will smile inside, knowing that by honoring this commitment to yourself, you'll feel nurtured, positive, and motivated to keep moving forward in a positive direction.

I encourage you to give each of the following steps a few days' practice before adding the next one. The goal is to make slow and easy changes that will last instead of attempting to follow another overly strict, change-everything-all-at-once diet (that's "die" with a "t") that you'll soon rebel against. Forget that. Yes, this method will take a few extra days, but so what? It's a lot easier to live with, and therefore you'll be able to enjoy sticking with it. For now, break out your journal, and take some notes as you read through the steps. Personalize them, use real names and real dates—and watch your customized food plan take shape!

A note on timing: The material that follows is exciting. It's the "user's manual" on how to develop a food plan that will get you to your healthy weight, and developing a food plan can actually be an enjoyable experience! But you may be wondering, "So when should I put this plan into action?" The answer is, as soon as you feel ready. Ideally this would be at least one month prior to surgery. The WLS program I went through, which is considered one of the best in the nation, had me practicing most of the guidelines I've listed here starting at least four to six weeks prior to surgery.

If you're post-op, you should receive specific guidelines from your WLS program on what to consume in the first weeks after surgery, then during the next one to three months, and finally during the following four to twelve months. Please follow these guidelines carefully, and don't stretch your pouch beyond its limit or you may suffer serious physical problems, anything from stomach pain and dumping to ending up in the hospital with a rupture.

If you are far enough post-op (six to twelve months) that you are able to consume most foods without any problems, then you may begin the following plan as soon as you can. Even if you don't feel ready right this minute, don't worry. There are methods included to help you *get* ready!

Step One (at least one week prior to start date)

- **Pick a date when you're going to start living this healthy, nurturing food plan.** Make it at least five to seven days from now. If you wish, have a last supper of your old favorite foods; say goodbye to them.

- **Talk to everyone in your life whom you might be eating with; tell them you're following a new "anti-diet" and to**

please support you in your efforts. When they ask what an anti-diet is and what kind of support you want, tell them an anti-diet is a nurturing, healthy food plan for life. Ask them to please refrain from offering you snacks. Ask those you live with to please keep any trigger foods out of sight so you won't be tempted. (As I said, my trigger foods are sweets, starches, and junk food.) Who knows, they may even join you on your new plan!

o   **In fact, it's a great idea to look around for someone who will follow this plan with you.** Even if they're not a WLS patient, they could still benefit from the food and exercise plan, and you could support each other. If you can't find anyone to join you, that's okay. It works just fine solo, too.

Step Two (at least five days prior to start date)

o   **Educate yourself.** Get all of the information you can on what constitutes a healthy nutritional plan for you. Yes, I know there are a million books and opinions on this subject. What has worked for me and many others is the basic plan recommended in Julia Ross's *The Diet Cure* and Barry Sears's *The Zone.* These plans emphasize a combination of proteins, heart-healthy fats, and a variety of fruits and vegetables. They also suggest avoiding sugar, white-flour products, caffeine, aspartame, and other less than healthy choices. *The Diet Cure* includes a helpful questionnaire that pinpoints the causes of your food cravings and emotional eating patterns and then recommends specific nutrional supplements that can eliminate your interest in trigger foods.

o   **Develop a list of your personal trigger foods, and either cut back on them or eliminate them from your food plan.** Once you've listened to the experts, then it's time to listen to your body. You'll know your trigger foods because you crave them above all others, and also because they may make you feel unwell—stuffy nose, headaches, stiff joints, swollen, irritable, sleepy, itchy. Do those sound like allergy symptoms? They are—and many people experience what health professionals call an "allergic/addicted" reaction to their trigger foods.

o **Find some physical activities you enjoy, and commit to doing them for at least half an hour, three to five days a week.** Mine are hiking in the forest, swimming, gardening, walking on the beach, yoga, and horseback riding. I'm still trying to appreciate going to the gym, but these other activities fill my heart and soul as well as move my body, so I tend to gravitate to them. Make your own list. And if you can find a friend to do them with you, all the better. My life is as busy as most people's, so whenever I can combine activities, like a visit with a friend and exercise, I do. It's a good idea to start the exercise plan right away, a few days before you begin the food plan. Enjoy it!

o **Get crystal clear about your nonnegotiables.** These are the aspects of your plan that you'll stick to no matter what. This is a very important part of your overall plan, and it may save you when things get rough. To help you discover what your nonnegotiables are, write your answers to the following questions in your journal:

My trigger foods are: _____

I'll handle these by ___ practicing zero tolerance / ___ having them once a week / ___ having them on special occasions / ___ other.

I will eat ___ meals and ___ snacks per day, at around _____ A.M., _____ A.M., _____ P.M., _____ P.M., and _____ P.M. I will stop eating by _____ P.M. (two or three hours before bedtime is recommended).

I'll find a fun way to exercise, _____ or _____, for at least ___ half an hour / ___ one hour / ___ other: _____.

I'll do my fun exercise ___ times a week, at _____ A.M./P.M., on the following days: _____.

Your list of nonnegotiables may not include all these things, but at a minimum it should include your trigger foods and exercise plan.

Step Three (at least three days prior to start date)

○ **Write down your general plan.** Include a page listing what foods you'll eat, a page listing what trigger foods you'll let go of, and a page listing the vitamins, other supplements, and amino acids you'll take. Be sure to include healthy foods you enjoy, and make a note of recipes that use them.

○ **Utilize vitamins, aminos, and essential fatty acids as an integral part of your food plan.** Did you know that a lack of certain nutrients can cause food cravings? For over a year into my recovery I was tormented by cravings for fried chicken, fried zucchini, fried just about anything. Once I learned that essential fatty acids such as omega-3 oils were missing from my diet, I began to use them on my salads—and the cravings disappeared. Again, *The Diet Cure* outlines a comprehensive plan for the use of nutritional supplements that can help you make a much smoother, easier transition. I include an abbreviated version of the plan in Appendix A, but I encourage you to read that book and apply what fits for you. (Appendix A also includes a sample grocery list and sample daily food plan.)

○ **Develop a clear idea of what your other relapse triggers (the nonfood ones) are, and plan ahead for them.** For example, many people, including me, report evening cravings as their worst trigger. I have an array of tools I use for this time of day. I take the amino acid L-glutamine around 5 P.M., and sometimes 5-HTP around 5:30. I have a healthy dinner just prior to 7:30 P.M., and I plan some kind of low-key activity for most evenings. Around 9 P.M., I'll have some herbal tea or sugar-free hot cocoa, write in my journal, visit with friends by phone, and maybe read a book. By 10 or 10:30, I'm ready for bed. If I can't sleep and still want to snack in the worst way, I'll take a hot shower or bath and have another cup of tea or cocoa, and usually that will do the trick. If you can plan some tools for use at *your* moments of temptation, it can really help you stay on track. Other examples of these kinds of triggers can include certain uncomfortable feelings, situations, or thoughts that make you want to deal with them by eating.

Step Four (at least twenty-four to forty-eight hours prior to start date)

o **Fill your kitchen with healthy foods that you enjoy.** Make a shopping list that is appropriate for where you are in your WLS process. Be sure that you also get plenty of water, vitamins, and minerals. I'd also suggest taking at least one amino acid, L-glutamine, to help with cravings. Look at the chart in Appendix A if you are having cravings and want to try some other amino acids to alleviate this and other symptoms.

o **Just before you start your plan, prepare some foods in advance.** This is for those times when you just can't wait. Many of us have found that when we're hungry or tired after a full day, that's the moment when we'll go for any food that's easy or convenient. God forbid I happen to be driving past a fast-food place right then! If something tasty is already made and waiting for you at home, it's much easier to hold out in moments like these. I'll typically spend a few hours once a week making chili, stew, quiche, or soup. Once it's made, I'll separate it into meal-sized portions, freeze some in microwaveable containers or baggies, and put the rest in the fridge. Then I'll chop up some lettuce and other veggies and separate them into meal-sized baggies. I might also prepare a salad-friendly protein source like chicken, tuna salad, egg salad, or soybeans, or my own sugar-free three-bean recipe. Sometimes I even make sugar-free desserts for those moments when I feel like I *have* to have something sweet. By planning and pre-preparing these foods, I can make sure to have something both yummy *and* healthy! Does this sound like a lot of work? It's worth it. For a few hours' effort once a week, I am provided with an abundance of fast, healthy, great-tasting food. Here's another lifesaver: Once you've gone to the effort of making all these great meals and snacks, take them with you when you're on the go! When I have my little cooler filled with healthy, yummy food, it's a snap to find something good in there rather than go buy a less desirable choice.

○ **On the day prior to your "start date," clean all the junk food out of your house, car, and workspace.** If there are places where you keep snacks (like in the car or in your desk at work), replace them with healthy (or at least low-impact) alternatives like sugar-free gum, sunflower seeds, or carrots.

○ **On the night before you begin, plan your meals for the following day.** Write down what you'll eat for each meal. It's helpful to include portion sizes as well. For example, a sample lunch might look like this: 3–6 oz. tuna salad with 1 tablespoon mayo and 1–2 cups chopped lettuce/shredded cabbage mix covered with 1–2 oz. feta cheese and 1 tablespoon dressing.

○ **At the end of each day, write down what you really did eat.** If you want to (and if you promise not to make yourself crazy over the numbers), tally up your proteins, fats, carbs, and calories for the day. There are several methods for doing this. I tally calories and protein, and document my exercise, too. This might seem like a lot of writing, but don't worry, it only takes five to ten minutes a day. Your local bookstore (I used Borders) will carry an array of little books for counting calories/protein/fat/carbs and measuring the caloric output of your exercise activities, and a similar array of mostly blank books for writing down your daily totals. You could also use your journal for these daily food and exercise records; that way, there are fewer books to worry about writing in, and if it's in the same journal as your daily feelings, you may see a connection between your emotions and your eating. If you're a computer whiz, there are free programs online that do these calorie/protein/exercise calculations for you. To make sure I was getting enough protein, I wrote everything down for my first six months post-op, and I still go back to doing it if I start to gain weight.

Some people suggest carrying your food journal around with you and writing everything down as you eat it, so you don't forget anything. If your memory of what you ate seems dim at the end of the day, this might be a good idea.

○ **Keep making these two lists**—the "before" plan, detailing what you will eat for the day, and the "after" list, of what you actually ate. Do this daily for at least a month, preferably longer.

○ **Once you have set up your plan, have set a date, and are ready to begin, relax and surrender yourself into following it.** The old diet mentality was all about fighting—fighting cravings, fighting with your body, fighting to stick to your diet while feeling irritable and deprived. No more! Think and talk positively about what you are doing. There is a certain relief and happy pride in yourself that comes when you are living in alignment with your goals. Feel this, focus on it, and share the feeling with those around you. If you can honor and relax into whatever feelings come up as you follow your plan day to day, you'll be surprised by how much easier this new strategy is than the old "fight with your body" diet mentality ever was.

Summary

1. Write down a healthy food plan for the day.

2. Prepare the foods you'll need for the day, and if you're leaving the house to go to work or elsewhere, consider taking a small cooler with you. Mine is filled with water, salad, baby carrots, hard-boiled eggs, string cheese, and fruit.

3. Plan a realistic time of day for exercise, and do it. "Realistic" means more than just a tiny slice of time in your busy day. It also means choosing a time when you'll have energy to follow through. If you can find a friend who'll join you, all the better!

4. Live your life, being kind and nurturing to yourself.

5. At the end of the day, write down what you did eat, and use your journal to write about (and let go of) any stress or other feelings or frustrating situations that may have occurred during the day. You can also use this time to plan the next day's food, so you will have it ready for the morning.

◎ Jennifer's Story

I met Jennifer, a twenty-seven-year-old artist, when she began attending my WLS support group. She was struggling with her old habits of snacking and being a couch potato, and she had regained some of the 125 pounds she'd lost after undergoing gastric bypass surgery the year before. Feeling frustrated with the conflicting advice of diet experts, she readily embraced the idea of formulating her own customized food plan.

She says, "I was excited to find something that wasn't just another cookie-cutter, one-size-fits-all diet. I really appreciated the fact that the food plan concept was developed by someone who had been through it herself, not some skinny doctor who didn't really understand. Since I've been using this food plan and found an exercise I really like—dancing—I've already lost ten pounds, and it's only been a month! I put on old Motown songs and just dance around the house when nobody's home—it's really fun. What I like the most is that it feels like a plan I can live comfortably with because it's based around my own strengths and weaknesses. Instead of feeling trapped by my cravings, I feel a sense of relief and freedom. It's working!"

Committing to Action

Throwing all of
your energy into
your goal —
a happier,
healthier you!

In my OEE classes we often joke about the "c" word, *commitment,* as though it were too hot to handle, too big to—well, to commit to! Why are so many people afraid of commitment? Maybe it's because every time we say an unqualified yes to one of life's choices, it usually means we are saying no to many others. We choose, but then we second-guess ourselves, wondering if the choice we made was the right one. Caught up in anxiety over this dilemma, we don't commit ourselves fully to the choice we made, delivering only a half-hearted effort because we still feel conflicted inside. Then we wonder why it didn't work out.

It's easy to dream about how great you'll look and feel when the weight comes off. The new clothes, the boost in self-confidence, the opportunities you've been wanting for years—all this is about to come true.

Or is it?

WLS can be the greatest transformation of your life—but *only if you commit yourself fully* to the changes that need to occur along with the surgery. You must choose to walk away from your old habits and self-image and embrace new ones.

During my career as a substance abuse counselor, I often had my clients complete a powerful assignment: writing their own eulogy. (A eulogy is a summary of a person's life, read at their funeral by a loved one.) Actually, I had my clients write two eulogies. The first was a hard-hitting, negative one, detailing how their funeral sermon might sound if they died of their addiction. It talked about their health problems, the loved ones they left behind, the dreams they left unfinished.

The second eulogy was a positive one, showing how their life and death might look if they took charge of their health right then and lived the rest of their life in recovery, healthy, happy, and free.

This process really brought home to my clients how each little choice, whether it was falling back into old patterns or stepping up to try something new, creates the tapestry of their lives.

Now it's your turn. I encourage you to give this next assignment your best, most sincere effort so that you, too, can truly begin to experience the feelings that will help you make a solid commitment to change.

ASSIGNMENT: "Dearly beloved,
We are gathered here today to mark the passing of ..."

Eulogy #1: Think realistically about where your life might go from here if you don't take charge of your health. If you stay on the same course you're on now, with your overeating and all of its consequences, how will your life, and death, turn out? Be detailed. Write from the perspective of someone who is reading this at your funeral. Who else would be there? What would they say about you?

Eulogy #2: Now think about what your life might be like if, from today forward, you were to choose to eat healthily, exercise often, and start living your dreams. What would the rest of your life look like? What might be remembered about you at your funeral? Who would be there? What would they say?

Once you've written your eulogies, find a supportive person to read them to. In addition, read them into the mirror, looking frequently into your own eyes. It might seem a bit silly, but trust me, it isn't. This ain't a game, folks. It's your real life we're talking about here.

Just prior to my surgery, I decided to have a "funeral" of my own ... for junk food!

The Goodie Bag Funeral

Inventory of items in the goodie bag:

- box of crackers
- one bottle of mayonnaise
- jam
- snickers
- four big pastries

- ○ brownies
- ○ potato chips
- ○ whipped cream
- ○ peanuts
- ○ peanut butter
- ○ pasta with cheese
- ○ macaroni and cheese
- ○ crackers and cheese
- ○ just plain cheese
- ○ one bottle of gooey sundae sauce
- ○ more stuff I can't, and mainly don't want, to remember

On the evening before my surgery, I needed to get rid of all the above food so I could come home to a "clean" house. Taken together, these items filled a pretty big bag. I took the goodie bag to a spot in the front yard that I can see from my living room window. I got a shovel and started digging. I had to dig a pretty big hole for all that food.

"What the heck are you doing?" my inner "gobble gremlin" asked. "This is a waste of time. Just put it back in the fridge for later," it pleaded, "or give it away to someone. Think of the waste!"

"Shut up, I'm busy," I said aloud, and kept digging. Yes, there probably were other things I could've been doing. I was getting on a plane for surgery soon, and I could've been packing or cleaning house. But there I was, burying a bag of perfectly good food (good? you saw the inventory). Luckily, my hedges are high so the neighbors couldn't see in.

I threw the bag into the hole, despite the protestations of my gobble gremlin. "Hey!" it cried, sounding strangely muffled. "Kinda hot in here, ya know? Can we talk about this?" After I'd covered the bag with dirt, I planted purple flowers on top, a hardy variety that is known to survive all sorts of toxic conditions. I took two wooden sticks and fashioned a cross, then found an old saucepan with a broken handle lying under some ferns (okay, so I don't have the tidiest yard). I used it to make a kind of headstone, which I set firmly into the ground above the flowers. I even said a little eulogy.

"Dearly beloved," I began.

"*MRBLLHMPHTTRT!!*" Something interrupted me from below the dirt, under the purple flowers. I ignored it.

"*I SAID, dearly beloved,* we are gathered here today to witness the untimely passing of an old friend, our gobble gremlin. Untimely because its suffering, and therefore our suffering, has gone on far too long. We'll mourn our friend for all the times it provided comfort, companionship, and relief. After all, it's human to go down the wrong road at times in search of these things. And, in its way, our old friend saved us when we needed saving, from things that were too terrible to face alone."

The neighborhood kids were beginning to gather behind the hedges as I waxed a little too loud in my eulogy. I'd better wrap this up.

"But we will also rejoice, because in its passing we are set free, to begin another life. A healthier, more open, fuller life. God bless us and amen."

I turned and walked into the house, ignoring a rustling noise coming from beneath the purple flowers.

"Yeah, I hear you, you devil," I said as I shut the front door. "I'm just not listening anymore."

ASSIGNMENT: How Committed Am I?

If you've completed the assignments up to this point, you've taken a look at your own history with food and weight, you've developed a nurturing food and exercise plan, and you've envisioned where you'll be if you *don't* get a handle on these issues. Doing the previous exercises can help move you forward into the most important phase of this plan. Now it's time to do more than think about it; it is time to live it. When you arrive at the commitment stage of the process, you must make a decision—or, really, a series of decisions.

Use your journal to answer the following questions:

- **Do I want freedom from food/weight problems *more* than I want to keep overeating?** This sounds simple, but it's not. Try to avoid a superficial answer here. Ask yourself on a deeper level than what would be required if you were simply starting another diet. What the question is really inviting you to consider is . . .

- **Am I ready to fully give myself, one day at a time, to a new way of dealing with food?** This is a radical shift from the diet mentality, which tells you just to go ahead and agree; it'll be over soon anyway. If you make a *real* shift, a real lifestyle change, you'll get real results. If you just do it halfway, you'll get the same thing you've always gotten. So give this question some genuine attention, and go deep with your response. Then make your decision.

- **Am I willing to face and deal with the feelings that may arise as I make these changes?** Food may have been a comfort, a relaxant, a lover, a friend. How will you meet the need for those things without it? You'll have a much easier time making this shift if you've already put into place a "full plate" of new tools when uncomfortable feelings come up. Whenever you let go of something that has filled a need in your life, it's important to bring in alternative sources of support. We'll discuss these tools in upcoming chapters.

- **Am I willing to set clear boundaries and priorities around this new way of life?** As we take a look at the different areas of your life that can either support or sabotage your food plan, one thing will become clear: You will need to set up some self-protective boundaries about what you will or won't eat, how you will or won't deal with the people in your life, how you'll handle social situations, how you'll deal with feelings. In the following chapters I'll give you some suggestions and tools, yet ultimately it will be up to you to set boundaries and keep them.

- **Am I willing to say goodbye to certain foods, maybe forever?** If you react to your trigger foods the way I do, you may have to cut them out of your life altogether. If so, consider doing some kind of a closure ritual, like writing a goodbye letter to your "gobble gremlin." It may sound silly, but creating some kind of finality will help you keep your commitment.

You may have noticed that the dreaded "c" word—commitment—is sprinkled liberally throughout these suggestions, and there is an important reason for this. Many of us have an irritating little voice in our heads that I call the "negotiator." The negotiator is like an unscrupulous lawyer looking for loopholes in your contract—it will do everything it can to sabotage your goals. It says things like, "One little piece of candy won't hurt—after all, you've had a hard day; you deserve it." Or it will say, "Why did I say I wouldn't eat French fries? I love French fries, and I've got to have some enjoyment in life. I can't just live on salads, right?" Or, "I'll just have this piece of cake now and exercise twice as long tomorrow." Sound familiar?

True commitment shuts down the negotiator. If I've got a plan for the day and I'm committed to following it, then there's nothing left to negotiate. It just is. And if you try this method, you'll find an unexpected gift that is a fringe benefit of your commitment: Once the negotiator is tied up and gagged, it will free up a tremendous amount of energy in your life. All the time I used to spend preoccupied with what I was or wasn't going to eat, all the mental and emotional energy I sacrificed to the negotiator to derail my goals—no more.

Here's one last tool that may prove very helpful:

- ○ **Spend a few minutes each day releasing your feelings in a journal.** Even if journaling feels unfamiliar at first, even if you are "too busy," or even if you're worried that someone will read it, this tool is so valuable that's it's worth finding a way to get past any obstacles and just commit to trying it for a month. I use my journal every night to write down what I really did eat that day and what situations or feelings came up and how I handled them, and then I record my food plan for the following day. Looking back over my journals has helped me to make and maintain major changes in my life.

Leading Up to Weight Loss Surgery

In the months prior to WLS, I went through about a million different emotions—hope, fear, concern, excitement, worry, you name it. At the same time, I had to go through a structured preparation process, sponsored by the medical team. These steps are meant to educate, inform, and support the preoperative patient in becoming as ready as possible when the time comes for the actual procedure.

If you have made the decision for surgery, you are probably getting excited and maybe even a little anxious about what it will be like. Your doctor will explain the surgical procedure itself to you and is also legally bound to present all the possible risks you may encounter. If it's a good program, like mine was, there will be a bariatric team who will advise and guide you through each phase of the presurgical process.

The best advice I received was also very simple. About six months prior to my surgery, I remember asking Candyce, our bariatric counselor, "What should I do to prepare myself for this surgery?" And she replied, "Right now you should start doing everything you expect to be doing after the surgery so you'll be familiar with it." Simple, but not necessarily easy!

Here are some of the guidelines most bariatric programs will expect you to follow:

o   Keep a food log of everything you eat. Count protein grams for sure, and count calories if you want to. (Again, many books and websites are available that can help you calculate the calories and nutrients in foods.) The intention here is not to become obsessive about counting, but to increase awareness about what you are doing.

o   Measure out one-ounce portions of liquids like soups and broths, and try them. This is the amount you'll be eating right after surgery and for the next several weeks as you recover.

o   Buy some small bowls and plates and begin to use them for your meals.

○ Practice chewing your food thoroughly and eating slowly. Many of the post-ops I've seen who endured problems like throwing up, dumping, or getting food stuck in their systems didn't do this.

○ Make an effort to eat according to the nurturing food plan you developed in Chapter 2. Although you won't be eating this way again until at least six months post-op, it makes sense to try to practice healthy eating now. Following a sound food plan will help your body be as healthy as it can be while you prepare for surgery.

○ Every day, take a multivitamin supplement containing double the RDA, with extra B vitamins and calcium.

○ Focus on eating at least sixty grams of healthy protein daily.

○ Focus on drinking at least sixty-four fluid ounces (one-half gallon) of water daily.

○ Try different protein drinks, powders, and bars to familiarize yourself with them—but don't buy a case of them! Your tastes will likely change right after surgery, and you don't want to be stuck with a big box of something that no longer tastes good to you.

○ Begin to move your body. Take walks, stretch, swim, do whatever you can to be physically active. Every time you exercise you will improve your breathing and circulation and strengthen your system—all of which are good preparation for surgery. Even if you have health challenges, work within your physician's guidelines to do *something;* simply moving around slowly in a swimming pool can help.

If you have other questions or concerns, the website www.obesity help.com offers lots of valuable information and support. Of course, please follow your own doctor's recommendations over and above anything I've said here; these are meant to be general guidelines only. Your specific health concerns and your doctor's advice about how to address them should be the primary recommendations you follow as you prepare for surgery.

What to Expect Before Surgery

You'll know a good WLS program by its thoroughness. The staff should put you through a series of tests and other requirements prior to surgery. Sometimes this will occur after you've been approved by your insurance; in other cases, the insurance company itself will expect you to complete the tests satisfactorily as part of their approval process. The presurgical requirements may include the following:

o   a heart stress test

o   a physical therapy session

o   a psychological testing and counseling session

o   extensive blood work

o   a session with a dietician or nutritionist

o   a session with a pharmacist to analyze your medications

o   support group sessions (required for pre- and postoperative patients)

o   any testing specific to your personal health concerns

o   a checkup plan for thirty days, ninety days, six months, and one year post-op, including regular blood work and counseling

If a bariatric program does not offer any preoperative counseling or testing, I would be very suspicious of its quality and of the ethics and skill level of its staff. Not everyone is suited for this surgery; some people have mental or physical health complications that make it unsafe for them. Statistics have shown that, after undergoing WLS provided by a program that does not offer any orientation beforehand or support system afterward—that is, a program that provides only the surgery itself—many people soon gain their weight back. As weight loss surgery becomes more popular, some surgeons, wanting to make a fast buck, are taking abbreviated courses in how to do it and then setting themselves up as "experts"—so beware. **Please, *please* investigate your bariatric surgery provider thoroughly before commit-**

ting yourself, as your life and your future are going to be in their hands. Ask questions, ask for references, and don't let your hurry to get skinny deter you from finding the best bariatric program and surgeon that you can.

Most of us go through a lot of soul searching before we even decide to have this surgery in the first place, and by the time we get to the doctor, we want things to hurry up already! Yet once we've passed the tests and are assigned a surgery date, all of a sudden the fantasy of getting thin is replaced by the realization of what's really involved—major surgery with a long recovery period—and we begin to get nervous.

This is perfectly normal, and the best thing you can do for yourself during the last few weeks or days prior to surgery is to use your support system to talk it out when you need to. Anyone whom you trust to be encouraging and positive can be part of your support team, including friends, family members, your doctor, or a counselor. Some WLS programs ask their post-op patients to serve as "WLS angels" (i.e., mentors or sponsors) to presurgical patients during the final days before and immediately after their surgery. When asked to be an "angel," I gave gifts, protein supplements, and moral support to newly recovering WLS patients—and I had "angels" who did the same for me. After all, no one else's reassurance is quite as helpful as that of someone who has been down the same road before you.

The Importance of Having a "Plan B"

What is a Plan B, you ask?

I wish I could just ignore this topic, frankly. But if I am to tell you all the important things about weight loss surgery, one of them is that you must make a "just in case" plan. Plan A is the one in which everything goes fine with your surgery and you experience a normal recovery process. Plan B is the one you formulate in case something goes wrong with your surgery and you need to designate someone to speak for you and carry out your wishes. This could happen due to a range of problems—from something as minor as your having to remain sedated for a few days, to something as serious as a coma or death. It's very rare for these kinds of complications to happen, and I know they're scary to think about, but it's better to think about them beforehand and to write your Plan B to cover any eventualities.

Think about the following as you draw up your Plan B:

o   Consider executing a power of attorney designating a friend or relative to make decisions on your behalf if you can't make them for yourself.

o   Decide how you want your responsibilities (bills, dependents, etc.) to be taken care of, in both the short and long term, if you are unable to take care of them yourself.

o   In the event of the worst-care scenario (sorry), you should write a will, including how you want your remains to be handled and any wishes you have for a memorial or funeral service.

I know, no one wants to think about these things, but they are important. Take the time to write about them, for both your own overall peace of mind and that of your loved ones.

What to Expect at the Hospital and During Surgery

Speaking generally, when you pack your bag to go to the hospital for surgery, expect to be there for at least three to five days. Most bariatric surgeons try to do the procedure laparoscopically, which typically requires a three-to-five day hospital stay. But this is not always possible, and your surgeon may need to do an open procedure, which requires a longer recovery period, usually including five to seven days in the hospital. The surgeon will also want you to return for follow-up at one week, two weeks, and thirty days post-op.

When you pack, you'll want to include—

- for women: at least two nightgowns, either short, sleeveless ones or the button-front kind. For men: button-front pajama shirts. Or you can just wear the fashionable and modest open-back gowns provided by the hospital

- a list of phone numbers of everyone on your support team

- slippers and a bathrobe for walks up and down the hall

- toiletries like toothpaste, toothbrush, lotion, etc.

- a few pairs of socks in case your feet get cold

- whatever medications you normally take (but check these out with your doctor first)

- a good book or videogame in case you get bored (I was too sleepy to read)

- at least two copies of your Plan B; give one to your doctor and one to your main support person

It's lovely if your support person can be at the hospital with you, but you'll be okay even if that doesn't work out. I flew alone to another island for my surgery, I came home alone, and I was fine. My best friend spent two nights at my house once I returned home, but it was more for moral support than because I really needed anything.

When you first wake up from surgery, you'll probably be groggy and medicated but relieved that it's over. Typically you won't be feeling any pain at this point, and very little afterward, too. You'll have lots of help and attention from the nurses, your support team, and your doctor. Sometime during the next twenty-four hours you'll be expected to go through a charming procedure called a "barium swallow," the most unpleasant part of the whole process, in my opinion. But it only lasts a few minutes, and it is vital.

The barium swallow allows the medical team to check for any leaks in your incisions that may have developed during or immediately following surgery. A leak is extremely serious and can cause severe infection or even death if not addressed quickly. Even if you had an open procedure and your surgeon tells you he checked visually for leaks, *insist on the barium swallow anyway!* I know of one patient whose surgeon figured that since she'd had an open procedure, he'd seen everything he needed to see and the barium swallow wasn't necessary. But he missed a leak, and she ended up with severe complications that landed

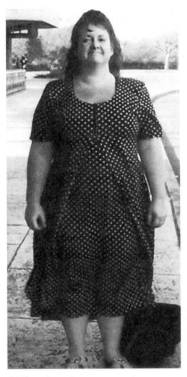

her in the hospital for months. So make sure they do the yucky but very important barium swallow.

Over the next few days, you will begin to be fed a clear liquid diet, and you'll be amazed at how little it takes to fill you up. Don't push it. Try to take small sips frequently, especially of water and protein. You'll also be expected to start walking, just a little at first, then up and down the halls, with or without the help of a nurse. Doing this is important because it helps prevent the formation of potentially serious blood clots in your legs following surgery. Nobody expects you to run a marathon, but a little walking now can prevent complications later.

You'll also be expected to prove

At the airport on my way to surgery

that your new, improved GI system is fully functional by having a bowel movement. By day three or four you may feel very ready to go home (I did), but you probably won't be considered ready for discharge until you can walk a little, eat and drink a little, and pee and poop a little.

In March of 2002 I flew to Oahu to have the surgery. During the week before I left, my friends kept asking me, "Aren't you scared?"— but I wasn't. I'd made my decision, I'd had months to prepare, and I fully believed this was God's path for me. So why worry?

But when the nurse drew my blood and I saw two big tubes being filled with it, I had to look away. I felt a little sick. Then, when they stuck me with their needles about ten times trying to find a vein for the IV and then started talking casually about putting the IV in my neck, I started to shake. I cried.

Then I woke up, and it was over. I had a sleepy, underwater feeling from the pain meds. Someone said to me, "Don't worry, it went great. You're in recovery now."

During the next few days I got to experience the safe, nurturing little world that is a hospital. Because I'd been Miss Super-Size portions all my life, I forgot about the reality of my tiny new stomach—until they gave me some little one-ounce cups and told me to use them to measure my intake. They wanted me to drink one fluid ounce over the course of every 30-minute period. That's two tablespoons, folks. *Are you serious?* I thought. *It's going to take me that long to drink that tiny cup?* But it did. And sometimes longer.

A big eater like I had been could wolf down vast quantities of food in a few minutes and barely realize they'd done it. Yet in the hospital I sent back meal after meal that had barely been touched, even though it consisted of just broth and Jell-O. I couldn't get it down. It was too much. Amazing. And, luckily, my appetite seemed to be gone along with it.

I spent three days in the hospital, during which time I received lots of nice phone calls and visits from people in my support group. Both my doctor and my surgeon came to check on me quite often, and the bariatric staff made sure I had no leaks in any of my incisions and that my GI system was working properly. On the fourth day I went home.

While going through my mail I chanced upon a copy of our support group newsletter. What I read astonished me. It contained a story about a woman who'd had complications from the surgery so severe that she'd been in a coma for a month, lost her speech and muscle functions, and took nearly a year to regain any normalcy in her life. I was floored, and humbled. The lady was someone I'd met at a group meeting, but I'd never realized how much she'd been through. Reading about her experience put everything into perspective. I was fine. My surgery had gone well. I said a little prayer, thanking God for bringing me this far.

What to Expect after Surgery

◎

For the first few weeks after you get home, be very gentle with yourself. Go slow, follow your doctor's instructions, and don't push yourself, *even if you feel fine*. I was in no pain, and I just had five small laparoscopic incisions. Sometimes I wondered if I had dreamed the whole thing! Until I tried to eat, that is. Then the reality of my situation was evident. I felt full after drinking just one ounce of liquid.

Most people describe their first few weeks after surgery as kind of surreal—they are moving slowly, being gentle with their bodies as they heal, and not eating. Or, at least, not eating very much. You will be on a clear liquid diet for the first couple of days, then a full liquid diet for the next one to two weeks. During this time you will drink tiny amounts of broth, juice, and protein supplements. From weeks three to eight post-op, you'll be on a pureed/soft food diet. One godsend for most WLS patients is that during this period, they aren't hungry. I've heard from WLS post-ops that the only time they craved food during the first weeks was if someone in their immediate environment cooked something they enjoyed and they could smell it or see others eating it. If you can avoid that situation, do.

Here are descriptions of the clear liquid diet, the full liquid diet, and the soft food diet:

Clear liquids include broths, such as chicken, beef, or vegetable, that contain nothing else. Sugar-free fruit juices are okay if diluted 50 percent with water. Diet beverages such as Crystal Light are also allowed. No sodas are permitted, not even diet ones; the carbonation is bad for

WLS patients. *Please be careful and go slow.* Remember, you have raw incisions on your stomach and intestines; they need to be stressed as little as possible while they heal. Visualizing these incisions helped me to remember to drink very slowly and to be very gentle with my GI system during the first weeks post-op.

Full liquids include all of the above plus cream soups, thin cream of wheat, thin sugar-free puddings, and thinly pureed foods, such as watered-down refried beans.

Soft foods include all of the above plus things like cottage cheese, tofu, soft fruits, applesauce, and sugar-free yogurt. Protein supplements are also critical at this stage, usually in the form of a clear or creamy protein drink.

A hint: Newly healing WLS patients generally don't tolerate foods like eggs, tuna, or even well-cooked vegetables. How will you know what you can tolerate? Stick to what has worked for other patients, and if a food is questionable, try just a little bit. If you can't tolerate it, you'll soon throw up. Not a lot of fun, but sometimes cautious experimentation is the only way to find out what you can and can't tolerate, besides checking with your doctor. Most WLS post-ops will throw up occasionally for the first few months, then less and less often as their system heals and they become accustomed to eating in this new way.

By week two or three, you can usually have mashed potatoes, and I was all excited to have one of my favorite binge foods legally. But the truth is, at this point you can eat and drink only a very small amount per day, so you have to budget. You're expected to take in sixty-four fluid ounces of water and sixty grams of protein daily, which frankly is far more than your system can probably tolerate at that point. So it makes better sense to stick with your proteins rather than waste that tiny amount of stomach space on empty carbs like potatoes.

After a month you'll have regained much of your energy, and you should be eating soft foods and slowly incorporating more normal foods as the weeks pass. Some patients throw up frequently at first;

some don't. I didn't. In fact, the only times I threw up were during my first month when I went out to dinner with friends and figured I could have "just a little" of what they were having. I spent the rest of the evening in the restaurant bathroom with my head in the toilet. Unpleasant and embarrassing.

My bariatric team strongly recommended that I take a full eight weeks off from work, and I got the okay from my employer to do so. But after one month at home I was feeling pretty good, plus I felt guilty about not being on the job doing my share. I made the mistake of going back to work too soon. I know of several WLS patients who did the same thing and regretted it. It's hard to explain exactly why you still get exhausted so quickly even six to eight weeks after surgery, but you do. And once you've already committed yourself to going back to your full-time duties, it may be too late to backpedal and say you made a mistake. If you can take a full eight weeks off, do it. Never mind if you're bored; this is your vitally important recovery time. It's all about making a good start on the rest of your life by healing fully before you get back into your everyday stresses.

Many patients, myself included, fail to realize how much time and energy they had previously devoted to food, to eating, or even to the comforting thought that food would always be their friend and solace. After WLS surgery that comfort is gone. In the first weeks post-op, when you're not eating and, hopefully, not working, you may find that there are a lot of feelings that come up and that you have a lot of empty time you need to fill.

When I arrived home from the hospital, I felt pretty good. All the dire predictions of what could've gone wrong never came true for me. By one week post-op, I was going for hikes in the forest with my dog, walking on my treadmill, cleaning the house—all much slower than before, but I was doing them. And I experienced no pain. The pain medication I took home from the hospital was ibuprofen, and I stopped using that after a few days.

So there I was at home, feeling pretty normal and wearing five small Band-Aids on my tummy. I wondered, *Is this all there is?* By the second week I was feeling like my everyday self, with a whole lot of time on my hands. Without the food to fill me and to ease my boredom and fear, I was like a sheepdog without any sheep. In short, I didn't know what to do with myself. And without my usual food party to entertain and numb me, a lot of feelings started to come up.

It's hard to write about those feelings. I felt a lot of grief over my divorce, which was barely two months old. A lot of love for my ex. A lot of anger and blame—for myself, then for him. I indulged in a lot of hamster-on-a-wheel mindtrips about how to repair the relationship we no longer had.

I knew that my addict mind, lacking food, was looking for another "fix." The gobble gremlin had returned, oh yes. He'd put on a suit and showed up at the front door trying to act like a gentleman and trying to make me turn my fix from food into love. But I could smell him coming. And whenever I'd given in to that urge in the past, whenever I'd tried to make something outside of myself responsible for my healing, it never worked.

So I ignored my inner addict and just felt the sadness and emptiness. What else was there to do?

Bottom line is, some feelings just need to be walked through, like a heavy rain. They don't need to be fixed, because they're not really problems.

In the past I'd worked on myself a little, then gotten overwhelmed, then slammed the lid shut again and dived back into food. And sometimes years would pass in guilty gluttony before I'd open myself up again.

But now I saw a ray of hope. Because I'd made the choice to have surgery and had finally stepped off the merry-go-round that many women spend their lives on—that of dieting, bingeing, and feeling bad about yourself. Believe me, a lot of energy can be sacrificed to this syndrome, energy that could be better used for so many other things. Like healing the past and letting it go, once and for all. Like really going for your dreams, big or small.

I knew that the surgery wasn't a cure-all to heal my old wounds, but it provided an opportunity to face everything, with no more "escapes" to tempt me. No booze, or drugs, or food, or even relationships. It was just me and God now, and no more distractions. It was like having a chance to come back to what's left of your home once a storm has passed, sift through the wreckage, and find something precious, something that miraculously escaped destruction.

And cherish it.

Overcoming Emotional Eating

*Ride the waves
of your feelings
instead of stuffing
them down*

Physical concerns are not the only ones that arise after surgery. Many lifelong overeaters don't realize how often they use food to cope with their feelings, problems, and relationships—until after surgery, when all those issues can come up with a vengeance.

The emotional challenges faced by the WLS patient are essentially the same as those faced by any other person dealing with food issues, except for the crucial distinction that the WLS patient is no longer physically able to use food to stuff their feelings. That means they must confront those issues immediately upon returning home from the hospital.

Over the first few months post-op, when you can only eat very little and the weight is coming off quickly, you may alternately feel exhilarated, exposed, thrilled, fearful, and vulnerable—especially if you've been big most of your life. Many WLS patients report going through a period of depression or experiencing mood swings after surgery. It is quite normal to sometimes wonder, "What the heck have I done to myself?"

This is a good time to join or start a WLS support group, get into counseling, or call on friends who will listen and understand. It is also a good time to write in your journal every day, using it to record your feelings and thoughts and to keep your food log. Instead of viewing this period as a roller-coaster ride you don't want to be on, see it as an opportunity to learn who you really are underneath the food. See it as a chance to get out of your comfort zone and try something new.

In the Cave

Two weeks after my surgery, I had the opportunity to attend an unusual spiritual retreat. A few of my friends had participated in a guided visionary journey called Breathwork that they described as being "like five years of therapy in a weekend." I wasn't sure that kind of thing was for me, but if I wanted to break out of old patterns after surgery, at least it was something completely new. My friends couldn't say enough good things about it, so I was persuaded to go.

Twelve of us attended the retreat, which was held at a fifty-year-old Zen monastery that was populated by Buddhist monks. The place was hushed and peaceful, full of greenery, with steep valleys stretching down to the ocean. The only sounds came from the surrounding streams and from the occasional bird in the bamboo forest above us.

The presenters were two very down-to-earth, likeable women, who met with us on the first evening for a briefing about what to expect. They described going into a trancelike state of awareness via deep breathing and very loud tribal music, and then having visions that were messages from the soul. They warned us that sometimes people became very emotional or very physical during their visions; their arms and legs might thrash about while they were in the grip of their waking dream. It sounded interesting and maybe a little dangerous, but I was willing to give it a try. I began to hope that maybe I would experience something big—transformational even.

Each of us was paired with a partner. When the session began, the deep thrumming of tribal drums and chanting filled the room. The volume was overpowering—I could feel the bass notes in my bones. But the music was strangely beautiful as well. The quality of the sound and its intense volume put both my partner and me in a trancelike state almost immediately. As I sat by my partner's side while she practiced the deep-breathing technique, part of me was watching over her, as I'd been directed to do, and part of me was far away, lost in a reverie. I was flying like a bird above the African savannah, soaring over golden plains and blue-green marshes. "I guess it's working," I thought. I closed my eyes and almost immediately saw—what? A vision? A daydream? I was awake, but it seemed as though I was having a very powerful dream.

At first, it was dark. Perhaps it was night. As the darkness slowly retreated, I saw a small campfire in a dry, rock-strewn clearing. There were mountains in the distance, and the air had the quality of the high desert, clear and razor sharp. Tiny stars far above barely punctured the blackness.

With the tribal music still pounding, suddenly a strange figure, a woman, leapt out from behind the rocks and began to dance around the fire. She wore a turbanlike headdress, with veils wrapped around her head like a mummy, hiding all but her eyes. Her long hair swung around her in knotted braids that looked something like dreadlocks. Plaited into them were artifacts and amulets—bits of bone and feather and colored stone that rattled and shook as she danced. Her body was clothed in an indigo coatdress and pants, and everything but her hands and eyes was completely covered.

As she moved in time to the fierce, primal music, three other similarly dressed figures appeared in the firelight and joined her. They danced with the same aggressive yet fluid cadence, and they looked at me as though they were trying to show me something or convey some meaning—only I couldn't make out what it was.

Finally the music shifted to a slower rhythm, full of long dissonant notes like a lonely wind sighing along the high desert plateau. The three other dancers were gone, and only the first one, whom I now recognized as a witch, remained.

She took me by the hand and led me into a deep crevasse among the rocks. Down and down we went along a narrow, winding path, through dark, echoing caverns. A soft yellow glow emerged from between the walls of stone, which opened up into a long, low cave. As we entered the cave my guide dropped my hand and silently gestured for me to take in the whole room.

We were in *my bedroom,* I now saw to my surprise. There sat my unmade bed from home, with my reading light and all of my favorite books piled beside it. Even my favorite cozy blanket and bathrobe lay across the foot of the bed. At first it was an inviting scene—until I looked up and saw the massive stone ceiling over the bed. It seemed to distend downward like rotten fruit, ready to split apart. It was an uncomfortable sight, off-kilter and out of balance.

It seemed that the cave was becoming smaller, claustrophobic; the cozy scene began to feel cloying and stagnant. All my little security blankets were right there waiting—everything I had always thought I needed whenever I retreated from the outside world after a breakup or a loss.

I looked again around the cave-room. It now felt uncomfortable, as if the air were growing thick, suffocating me with each breath I tried to take. I looked at the witch and made a panicky motion for her to get us out of there. She held out her hand to me, her expression inscrutable behind the headdress. When we reached the surface, she stared at me again with narrowed eyes, looking like a fierce, silent bird of prey.

I understood perfectly what I had been shown. In the cave was my life, or at least the part of it that had become so stagnant. Over many years of hiding from the hurts of living in the world, I had built that subterranean room, its walls buttressed by denial, despair, and, of course, food.

Escaping to my haven had become a destructive habit; I no longer needed a reason to hide—I would just do it. It was a place for dreaming, reading, eating, sleeping—and it was fraught with the urgency of repressed creative power ready to burst forth but always stalemated by overeating.

I didn't like what I saw, but I understood. This was where I'd lived when denial took me over, where I pretended that everything was okay when it wasn't.

The vision faded as the music changed again, but the eyes of the witch stayed with me. Later, when it was time to draw what I had experienced, she was the first image I drew. I also painted a softly lit cave with a cozy-looking bed pushed against a lowering rock ceiling. I colored its walls in a heavy, dark pastel to convey the room's thick, oppressive atmosphere. The drawing was a concrete reminder of what I took away from that weekend: the realization that sometimes a supposed hideaway can become a prison, and that the longer I put off facing my life, the heavier those walls would become.

Leaving Denial Behind, Embracing Clarity

You may find that once you put food in its proper place, that of nutrition, many unexpected feelings will start to surface. Some of them will be wonderful: a sense of pride in your decision and in your day-by-day accomplishments as you take better care of yourself. You'll be clear-headed, confident, and strong. This clarity will energize you, but it will also *sensitize* you—to situations and emotions you may have been suppressing.

Feelings of anxiety and vulnerability, as well as occasional mood swings, are also often reported by people who have stopped using food to cope. These emotions can seem overwhelming, and they can trigger a return to overeating. A better choice is to seek the underlying message that the feelings are trying to send. There are always good reasons why difficult emotions come to the surface.

Dealing with our emotions will be a big theme throughout this book. It's important to remember that our old ways of using food to suppress, numb, or nurture our feelings was not a sin, a defect, or a sign of moral weakness. We may have used food to cope with situations or emotions that were painful or overwhelming without even knowing that other ways to handle them existed.

These coping methods became habits, and those habits have now *outlived their usefulness.* Changing habits may seem insurmountable at first, but habits are learned, and they can be unlearned. How? By learning to understand our feelings and what they are trying to communicate to us. By learning what we *really* need.

There are several layers of feelings that may have been suppressed by using food. There are feelings arising from normal everyday stress as we face the ups and downs of living. Underneath these, often there are knotty problems that we keep avoiding, and underneath these, there may be old patterns of relating to others and ourselves that got us into these thorny situations in the first place. Often we have beliefs about ourselves and the world that we've been carrying around for years without realizing it.

If we are to rid ourselves of the habit of overeating, then we'll have to shine a light on these beliefs and ask ourselves, "Is this belief helping or hurting me? Is it always true, or could there be another way of looking at the situation?"

Imagine an iceberg, only a small portion of which is visible above the ocean's surface. The vast bulk of it is hidden underwater. Our layers of suppressed feelings function in much the same way. We know we're supposed to show only so much of how we really feel—just enough to make ourselves and others comfortable. So we shove the rest of our emotions down, often before they are felt or processed.

When we do this, a backlog of feelings starts to pile up. Over time, the backlog gets heavier and heavier, and if we use food to keep it all stuffed down, most likely *we* are getting heavier and heavier, too!

Take a look at the diagram below, which represents how layers of feelings and old traumas get buried. Has stuffing feelings with food been a problem in your life?

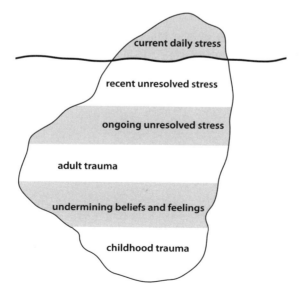

Our feelings operate like an iceberg, with many layers under the surface

Let's consider these feelings as they came up for a client of mine, Patricia.

Current daily stress: Patricia, a single forty-one-year-old social worker, was working full-time as a crisis counselor and taking care of her elderly mother at home. To make extra money, she was often on call at work, covering the crisis hotline from her cell phone. As she awoke each morning, her mind immediately began going over the upcoming day, and she often rushed out the door carrying only a cup of coffee, her daytimer, and her cell phone. Around noon she'd start feeling weak and hungry, grab a quick fast-food meal, and eat it in the car on the way back to the office. By the end of the day she was usually exhausted, but she'd fix dinner for herself and her mother before she collapsed in front of the TV. While the only free time in her busy day slipped away, she watched mind-numbing sitcoms and snacked on cookies or chips, letting the sweet taste and a full belly substitute for real nurturing in her life.

Recent unresolved stress: Patricia had been working as a crisis counselor for ten years, and the toll the job took on her emotionally was reaching critical levels. She wanted to quit, but because she was overweight she felt insecure about the possibility of getting another job. She repeatedly asked her brothers and sisters to help with caring for their mother, but they always said they were too busy. "Mom needed the help," Patricia said, "and nobody else was stepping up to the plate, so I just did it."

Ongoing unresolved stress: Patricia longed for a family of her own. She especially wanted a loving partner who would support her through the uncertainty of changing jobs and possibly putting her mother into long-term care. But she was so busy that she never had time to go out and meet men. Furthermore, she struggled with hypoglycemia, obesity, bouts of depression, and insomnia. "I felt there was far too much wrong with my life for anyone to want to get involved with me," she said.

Adult trauma: About two years prior to taking my OEE (Overcoming Emotional Eating) class, Patricia ended a five-year relationship with a man she had hoped to marry. "Mike was a charming, wonderful man in some ways," she recalled, "but he also had a temper, which got worse when he drank. For a long time I told myself that we could work it out. He was always sorry after a blowup, but eventually I became so mentally and emotionally drained that my only comfort was to eat late at night after he'd gone to bed. Over the years, my overeating and his drinking both got worse. When my mom's health deteriorated to the point where she needed someone to live with her, I saw it as an escape, and I took it. Since then, I've been pretty leery of relationships."

Undermining beliefs and feelings: Patricia was secretly relieved that she was too busy to go out socially. Because she was overweight, she didn't think any man would want her. And although she resented her job, and at times resented her invalid mother, at least part of her felt appreciated and wanted when she was caring for someone else's needs. "For a long time I believed I couldn't do any better, couldn't get an easier job or have a decent relationship because of my weight," she said. "Maybe that's because I didn't think I was worth much to begin with."

Patricia admitted that she may have been keeping extra weight on as a way to avoid men. She said, "Instead of having to *say* no, I can *be* no, to keep them from even making the first move. But it gets lonely. I really don't want to spend the rest of my life this way."

Childhood trauma: Patricia's father passed away due to alcoholism when she was thirteen, and afterward her mother worked two jobs to support the family. Because her father had been a religious man, the family never discussed how his drunken rages and frequent absences affected them. As the eldest daughter, Patricia was expected to go to work and help the family, so at sixteen she began working as a nurse's aide in a local hospital. By the time she was twenty-five and her youngest sibling was graduating from high school, Patricia found herself ingrained in a lifestyle that was difficult to break away from: helping others.

During her time in the OEE class, Patricia learned to make connections between the painful events in her past, her poor self-image, and the reasons she'd been overeating.

She utilized a high-protein, low-carbohydrate diet to alleviate her depression and hypoglycemia. As her physical symptoms diminished and she gained more energy and self-confidence, she was better able to practice setting boundaries at work and eventually enlisted her family's financial help in hiring a part-time nurse to assist in caring for her mother.

All of a sudden she had the free time and energy she had always wanted, which led to some surprising discoveries. "At first I was at a loss—scared, just floating around in space," she said. "In all my adult life I'd never had the freedom to focus on what I really wanted. And now that I had it, I didn't know what to do with it! But with some encouragement from my counselor and supportive friends, I began to participate in life. I went back to school and got involved with a local environmental group that went for nature hikes on the weekends. As I got busy doing things that nurtured my soul, I obsessed less and less about food. My extra weight slowly fell away, and I began to like myself inside and out."

Coming Out of the Fog: Finding Your True Self Beneath the Food Trance

◎

From Patricia's story we get a glimpse into some of the complexities you may encounter as you begin dealing with the hows and whys of overeating. To fully address her dilemmas regarding food and body image, she had to courageously explore many other areas of her life: her thoughts and beliefs, her family history, her relationships, and, of course, her eating habits. She had to take a look at both the payoffs she received from overeating and the more obvious problems it caused.

ASSIGNMENT: Uncovering Your Own Iceberg

Draw your own "iceberg," and label it with the layers of feelings shown in the diagram on page 73. Leave enough space in each layer to answer the following questions in some detail:

1. **What are the current daily stresses in my life?** (List three major ones.) Am I making time for enough rest, nutrition, and exercise? What would I have to do differently in order to make this time?

2. **How well do I process my feelings?** Do I stuff them down or express them in a healthy way? What am I afraid might happen if I fully expressed my feelings?

3. **What are the recent or ongoing problems in my life?** Do I have a relationship, a job, or other life situations that I wish were different? What underlying fear has kept me from dealing with these situations?

4. **What painful events have happened in my adult life that may be holding me back now?** Could my food/weight issues be an excuse for "hiding out" instead of risking rejection?

5. **What undermining beliefs or attitudes do I have that might be sabotaging my goals?** What did I learn while growing up, about myself or about life, that might be getting in my way?

6. **What experiences did I have as a child or young adult that may have made me fearful instead of confident?** How have these old messages been reinforced in my adult life?

You may be surprised to discover how old beliefs and feelings can affect your life today. Below is an account of how I addressed an old emotional issue following WLS.

Retiring Xena

By the fifth week after surgery I was back at work, living my life, and down twenty-five pounds. I knew I had some important choices to make. I could stay in my familiar but stagnant cave or venture out and participate in the world again, with all its risks and joys.

So many opportunities presented themselves! I could go to a yoga class, work on my paintings, see a movie with a friend, go to the beach. Everything was about going going going, and I had to frequently remind myself that I still needed time for my inner work, to help my head and heart catch up to my body. I was praying every night, writing in my journal daily, and going to therapy once a week.

My therapist, Jenny, and I talked about how a person's attitude creates their reality. For most of my life, I'd adopted the attitude of a soldier on active duty. I felt I always had to be strong. I never wanted to let anyone down. Sometimes, trying to hold everything up and keep it from crashing down around me felt like an enormous task. Everyone knows that in a crisis you just take action and save the feelings for later. But crises aren't supposed to happen every day. We aren't meant, as human beings, to *stay* in that keyed-up fight-or-flight mode evoked by crisis.

As a kid I had to be vigilant, watching for any situation in which the tension between my parents might spiral out of control. And when it did, I'd step in and do anything I could to distract them from getting into a big fight, even if it meant they would turn their rage on me. So, by necessity, I toughened up. I called it "standing up for myself," and if it had been only that, maybe it would've been okay. But it's never easy to gauge the trajectory of harsh words spoken in rage. By the time I was eighteen I felt like a seasoned soldier—one who had fought so many campaigns that my weapons and armor had never been retired. Familiar as skin, they were always ready to defend me from any threat, real or imagined.

Trouble is, there's really no place for a soldier in peacetime.

That day in therapy the proverbial lightbulb went on. "I get it!" I said to Jenny. "There's a part of me that's like Xena, Warrior Princess!" (Xena is the heroine of a popular TV show in case you've never seen it).

"Yes, and you must have created her when you were very young," Jenny replied. "You should honor her, and thank her for all her years of faithful service." I mulled this over, imagining the TV Xena with her sword and shield, snarling as she dove into the fray, vanquishing piles of sweaty, hide-covered men. Maybe holding on to this part of me wasn't so bad after all.

"And maybe," Jenny continued, puncturing my fantasy, "you should think about retiring her. You have grown into a smart, independent woman. Maybe you don't need her to protect you anymore. Maybe she's tired of fighting."

I nodded quietly, remembering the painful process of constructing of my own personal Xena. In my family, doing well was taken for granted, while anything less was pointed out, picked on, and shamed. In my childhood efforts to combat the constant criticism, I began to develop my shield and weapons. I went from getting A's in school to cutting class every day, and from being basically a meek kid to one who fought back. When I wasn't fighting I hid behind my armor of drugs and food and cigarettes and TV. I learned how to keep the scared kid concealed behind the tough one, and as I thought about it now I knew she'd served me well.

I kept her with me for so long that I forgot there was any separation between us. Whenever any threat, real or imagined, presented itself, the sword flew out and there was my Xena, lopping off heads before I could even think about it. Unfortunately, sometimes they turned out to be the heads of my friends, or of loved ones. Relationships suffered and sometimes disintegrated because of my anger and fear.

Even though I'd spent years creating a safer, calmer life for myself, making a pleasant home instead of a threatening one, no one had sent a message to the front lines telling Xena to stand down. She was still protecting the child I'd been long ago.

It was, indeed, time for her to retire.

I took some quiet time that night, said a prayer, and summoned up this protector from my childhood. To my surprise, she didn't protest when I told her that I no longer needed her. Instead, I heard her sigh in resignation and relief. I heard the swoosh of metal as she slid her sword into its sheath.

"But listen," she said in her rough voice, "you know I'll still be here for you whenever you need me, for anything you can't handle, any time at all."

"I know, and thank you," I replied. "But I think God and I will take it from here. I'll call on you if I really need to, don't worry."

We gave each other a nod of mutual respect and said goodbye.

Some Solutions: Finding Support Inside and Out

◎

Hopefully answering the questions posed in the iceberg exercise will give you a better understanding of where you've come from, what you learned there, and why you do the seemingly contradictory things you do—like overeating when you want to lose weight! Although understanding the problem is very useful, you will need to add positive tools for change if you are to move forward.

In the past, when I'd had a rough day I would fantasize about what yummy thing I was going to eat that night. Often I'd stop at the store on the way home and eat my "treat" in the car. Now, I consciously turn my mind to other ways to relax. I may plan what great music I'm going to listen to while taking a hot bubble bath. As the bathtub is filling, I'll light some candles and incense, creating a soothing environment for my body, mind, and spirit. I have learned to "crave" my warm bubble bath, and now I look forward to it as much as I used to look forward to food!

Here are some important tools to support you as you work through stress, past or present:

- Bring nurturing people, places, and habits into your life.
- Call a friend (a gentle, positive one).
- Play with children.
- Write in your journal.

o   Visit with someone you love.

o   Rent a funny movie (I like watching "chick flicks").

o   Enjoy some dog or cat therapy if you have pets (hugging your kids is great, too).

o   Get a good massage.

o   Pray or meditate for fifteen to thirty minutes with soft music playing in the background.

o   Sip a soothing cup of tea or clear soup.

o   Read a good book.

Of course, having a nutritious meal is certainly a good option, too, if that is what's called for. There's nothing wrong with enjoying food in its proper time and place.

In my experience as an addictions counselor and a WLS patient, emotional upset and/or a lack of nurturing are two of the primary reasons why many people overeat. Please give special attention to your own needs in these areas. They may prove to be key for you, too!

Support Groups

I've been facilitating support groups for over fifteen years, and I never cease to marvel at their effectiveness. They are the foundation of the twelve-step philosophy, which has helped millions of people worldwide let go of their addictions. An indefinable power to persevere comes from listening to and sharing with one's peers, and I highly encourage you to try it.

A few months after my surgery, I began leading a support group for WLS patients, both those who'd had the surgery and those who were considering it. The group was sponsored by a hospital, and it was my job to provide information about the surgery in a neutral manner, neither promoting it nor advising against it. "Just tell the truth about your own experience," they said, which was easy enough to do. As the group members got to know one another, we all agreed that sharing our ups and downs with others who had been through the same thing provided us with a source of reassurance and unexpected strength.

When we talked about the reasons why we overate, we found that we all had a hard time setting boundaries—we didn't know how or when to do it. Some group members didn't even know what boundaries were. I described the problem by saying, "It's when you know you ought to say 'no,' but you don't. It's when the people in your life expect too much of you, or you never have the time or space to nurture yourself, because you're always busy taking care of everybody else." Several heads in the room were nodding, and one lady spoke up.

"Between my boyfriend, my kids, and my job, it seems like I never stop," she said. "My boyfriend is really worried about me having the surgery—not because of *me*, but because then he'll have to watch the kids! The doctors have said they are going to meet with him to try to help him understand. But I don't know. The way things are now, I baby him. I do everything for him just like his mom used to. And if I have the surgery, I know I'll have to cook healthier and go out without the kids to exercise. I don't know if he'll put up with it."

"You'll need to start taking care of *yourself* for a change, right?" I said. She nodded ruefully, and said, "Right. And I hope I can be strong enough to really do it, because a lot of my family members have had strokes or heart attacks, and many died around the same age I am now, from things related to their weight. I want to be there to see my kids grow up." Everyone agreed, and gave her a few words of encouragement.

Another woman chimed in, "My husband is really good and is understanding, but for me, it's my sister. She drops her kids off at my house almost every day with the excuse 'You'd better take them, or I'm going to kill them,' and out the door she goes. Now, I love my nieces and nephews, but that's not the point. She acts like I have no life of my own, that all I ever do is cook for everyone and watch their kids. But you know what? They're her kids, after all. My kids are grown. It's time I started living my life."

We couldn't always find ready-made solutions for these concerns, but we did listen and care. What was evident was the value of the encouragement and empathy that we provided for each other—which was especially valuable for those who had a hard time getting it anywhere else.

If you are hoping to make changes that are lasting, statistics show that the people who keep their excess weight off over the long term are those who participate in some sort of support group. These folks have the best results. Therefore, I encourage you to consider joining a support group of people who are committed to dealing with their chronic overeating. If you can't find one, you can access the hundreds of WLS support groups online, or you can start your own! Guidelines for doing so are provided in Appendix B.

How to Retrain Your Brain

*Choosing
nurturing thoughts
over negative ones*

Many cultures and spiritual traditions have emphasized the importance of our thoughts and beliefs in determining everything from our attitude, to our bank balance, to our pants size.

Why do we think the way we do? In most cases, the way we think has been formed by three things: our family, our society, and our personal experiences. We make decisions about how we see ourselves and the world based on these "filters." Let's talk about each one in turn and see how they may be helping or hurting our goals in the area of food and body issues.

Family Influences
◎

Did you grow up in a home where you were encouraged to be yourself, were supported in expressing yourself, and were lovingly helped to grow into the unique and special person you are? Or were you, like many of us, told, "Stop that," or "Be quiet," or "You'd better not cry or I'll give you something to cry about!" Our parents did the best they could, and no doubt they gave us many good qualities to take into adulthood. However, they may have also instilled their own fears, insecurities, and faulty beliefs in us, at an age when we were too young to know better than to accept them.

For example, many parents who lived through the Great Depression in the 1930s (a time when many people were broke, unemployed, and had very little to eat) became somewhat fearful and conservative as a result. They may have passed their fears on to their children and grandchildren. A person who comes from this kind of background might take on these "family fears," becoming very insecure and afraid to try anything new because their parental programming told them not to. An Ivy League family, in which generations of offspring have gone to college, tends to continue producing college graduates; likewise, families in which generations have lived on welfare often perpetuate this difficult cycle. No one is forced to follow the family pattern; it's just another example of how the environment we grow up in exerts a strong influence on our lives. Does this mean that the college-bound family will never produce a "black sheep" or that the welfare family will never produce children who will rise above their roots? Of course not. They are free to change their family pattern at any point. And so are we.

For those of us dealing with food issues, the contrast between the voice of our inner spirit, which calls us to be free and to move forward, and the repressive voice of our old family filter may cause us to overeat repeatedly instead of facing and dealing with this conflict.

Societal Influences

We are bombarded daily with so much media persuasion—from TV, radio, and newspapers, to magazines, websites, and billboards. It's everywhere, and it is relentless. You might say that you know better than to believe in any media hype, and I'm sure you do. Yet if you watch TV or listen to the radio, then these carefully calculated messages wash over you day after day.

It's all geared to make us think we're never good enough the way we are—that we don't quite measure up (but if you buy their product, then you'll be fabulous, right?). Perhaps even against our better judgment, we begin to wonder if we're thin enough, young enough, rich enough, whatever enough! If you're not, the message says, then you'd better get with the program, because otherwise you're gonna miss out on the good things in life.

This way of seeing the world keeps us looking for our next "fix," whether it be falling in love, winning the lottery, or losing the weight. The happiness and satisfaction these products are supposed to give us always exist somewhere out there, never right here.

The diet industry, like most other commercial interests, has taken advantage of this way of thinking by focusing on our insecurities about

weight and body image. The current cultural obsession with slimness may seem like the way it's always been, but, in fact, ideas of beauty have shifted throughout history. The "ideal" body has changed several times, even in the last seventy-five years—from the slender, boyish "flapper" look of the 1920s to the curvier, full-figured body type admired in the 1940s and 1950s. Even in the early 1960s, a fuller figure was considered ideal. Perhaps you've heard the often-quoted statistic that Marilyn Monroe was a size fourteen, and many popular stars from her era, such as Ava Gardner and Jayne Mansfield, were a similar size. What changed? How did we become the skinny-crazed society we are today?

Some fashion historians say it happened because the curvaceous runway models of the 1950s got more attention than the clothes they were wearing! According to some accounts, fashion designers said, "If we use skinny models, then our customers will focus on the clothes, not the girls." Beginning in the 1960s with the famous model Twiggy, the women presented in the media became progressively slimmer and younger, until by the 1980s and 1990s the new "ideal" body type, at almost six feet tall and weighing 110 to 120 pounds, was a nearly impossible goal for most women. If you take into consideration current imaging technology, then what was nearly impossible moves even further out of reach. Why? Because nowadays almost every photo you see in the media has been edited or enhanced by computer. Even the slimmest supermodels, once they've been photographed for an ad, have their already lean upper arms and thighs trimmed further by a computer-editing program. Several recently popular TV shows promise to create the ideal beauty via plastic surgery, displaying their "before and after" models for us. But such transformation can only be had for a big price.

Add to this recent advancements in plastic surgery techniques and easily obtainable credit card financing and you have millions of perfectly normal women running to the plastic surgeon, or purchasing the latest diet book, pill, or strategy.

The problem is that the ideal they are going for—the ideal that women everywhere are beating themselves up over and which they can't seem to achieve—*was never real in the first place. It was created by the powers in the fashion and diet industries, powers that don't care whether or not you hate your body; they just want to sell you something.*

But the beauty and fashion industry can't take all the blame for our culture's worship of thinness. A vicious, barely hidden fat prejudice exists that many of us fall prey to, buying into the belief that overweight people are disgusting, lazy, and sloppy. Again, though it may seem as if society has always been this way, it hasn't. Fat prejudice is a phenomenon of our modern times and has no more basis in fact than racism or sexism. Let's look at institutionalized sexism as an example of what I'm talking about. From biblical times right up to the 1900s, many volumes, often written by doctors, psychiatrists, and other respectable authorities, were published that presented supposed "facts" about the physical, mental, and moral inferiority of women. Today, of course, these books and their authors would be laughed at (or cursed at). No one would take them seriously. Modern Western society no longer accepts this overt prejudice against women. Yet most folks don't question their fat prejudice.

Many people are uncomfortable admitting that they think fat people are disgusting. Instead, they'll say they are worried about the health problems associated with being big. Everyone agrees that extra weight brings terrible health risks. Where did these beliefs come from? From doctors, who only care about our good health and welfare?

Actually, no. The idea that health risks increase when we put on even a few extra pounds originally came from the health insurance industry. We all know that the way insurance companies make money is to sell you a policy based on dire predictions of what *might* happen, then limit their obligations as much as possible to avoid having to pay out claims if anything *does* happen.

With regard to health and life insurance, companies wanted to reduce the size of the group of people who had "normal health" because folks who fell into that category would pay the lowest premiums. Having any health problems or risks would mean that a customer would have to pay more for insurance. The more issues that were considered a potential health problem, the more money the insurance companies could make.

All of a sudden, carrying a few extra pounds became a "health risk," requiring the bearers of that additional weight to pay more for insurance. Doctors on the payroll of insurance companies created the first ideal height/weight tables, which arbitrarily decreed how much men and women *should* weigh. They began to advocate for the lower body weights, citing heart problems, high blood pressure, and other health issues as risks if a person weighed even ten or fifteen pounds above the "ideal."

But not all the predictions of heath problems associated with being overweight have turned out to be true. Exercise physiologist Glenn A. Gaesser, Ph.D., in his book *Big Fat Lies: The Truth about Your Weight and Your Health,* cites a more recent, equally compelling body of medical research that refutes the idea that being overweight automatically means sickness or disease.

I encourage everybody, including you, my dear reader, to think for yourself, investigate for yourself, and educate yourself on the important issues of our day, including the issues of weight and body image. You may be surprised by what you find. And if you should learn, as I have, that our societal epidemic of fat prejudice is *not* always based on health—that sometimes, it's one more example of greedy corporate interests trying to sell you something—perhaps you can feel some compassion for the next obese person you see. And have some compassion for yourself whenever you think you don't measure up to the hype. Don't buy it!

Personal Experiences

◎

Whether life has handed you mostly flowers or mostly lemons—happy times or hard times—those experiences are bound to have an influence on how you think. Sometimes life events were of our own choosing, and sometimes they seemed to come out of nowhere. Often our family "filter" has a big impact on how we see these situations, but ultimately it is up to each of us to choose how we want to view them. "Your attitude creates your reality" is one of those trite but true New-Age quips—and often our *thinking* is what creates our attitude in the first place! Therefore, it is to our benefit to get clear on what is going through our minds, to determine whether it is helpful or hurtful to who we want to be, and to choose accordingly.

How Your Biochemistry Affects the Way You Think

◎

It's common sense to acknowledge that if we practice good nutrition, get enough rest, and get at least some regular exercise, we will think more clearly and feel better than if we run on too little sleep and lots of stress, carbs, caffeine, or sugar. Over the past twenty years, however, significant scientific research has confirmed many aspects of the body-mind connection. Some of the traits once ascribed to our personalities, such as being outgoing or shy, assertive or insecure, have been shown to be based in our genetics and in the chemical messages transmitted by the brain.

More and more scientific studies are bringing home the point that some, and perhaps a great deal, of what we think and feel is influenced by what goes on in our body (and vice versa). For example, did you know that certain chemical imbalances in the brain can cause worry, obsession, and self-destructive thinking? Some of us have deficiencies in our brain or body chemistry that cause us to have these symptoms, or to be tired all the time, or to be anxious all the time.

And many of us, faced with these difficulties, will "self-medicate" with food to try to deal with the problem. The afternoon pastry and coffee when you'd rather take a nap, or the bowl of cereal and milk late at night because it helps you get to sleep—these are examples of how we may unconsciously gain weight when we're really trying to address a different problem: the way we think or feel. If you take care to follow a diet that includes plenty of protein, fresh vegetables, and fresh fruits, and you get regular exercise and enough rest, you'll most likely be pleasantly surprised by how well your brain chemistry is regulated and, therefore, how much your thinking and your moods are improved.

Breaking the Fantasy
That when You're Thin
Everything Will Be Wonderful

Yes, I know, your rational mind knows better than to believe in fantasies. But let's not forget all the cultural programming and the media brainwashing that says losing weight *does* work, you *will* get the guy, get the job, get the validation you've always deserved—once you're thin enough. Fact is, when and if you lose the weight, you probably will feel better. You probably will get more attention and compliments. And—you'll still be you, with your same life, your same choices, and all the same familiar comforts and flaws you had before. In other words, losing weight can improve your life in general, and it may provide more opportunities in love and work, but it's unrealistic to think it will magically solve all your dilemmas. There will still be plenty of opportunities to challenge your mind, your heart, and your problem-solving skills!

Here's how I handled some of those challenges:

In my second month after surgery I was given an opportunity to show my paintings in a local art gallery. This was a small miracle considering the fact that I'd never developed a complete portfolio. Every time I'd try to paint, the demons of doubt would close in, and I would hide behind food again. But this time, I couldn't! Thanks to the surgery, I had to face this scary and wonderful opportunity head-on, and it turned out to be a gift. It gave me a creative focus that I'd always said I wanted, and I threw myself into it.

I cut back on most of my socializing and focused on my painting. I worked, came home, and painted. I began to feel a pride in myself that I hadn't felt in a long time. By the time I'd finished my first collection, I was nearing the end of my third month post-op, and I'd lost fifty pounds. I saw this as a transfer of energy. Where once there had been fifty extra pounds on my body, now there were these paintings, big as life, hanging in a gallery. It was as if I'd taken the energy right off of my body and injected it into my artwork.

They say fat deposits in the body are a form of stored energy. During all the years when I stayed stuck in a rut and ate to cover the pain, the stored fat that resulted was a form of stagnant energy. And now, thanks in part to the surgery, I was finding the courage to battle my demons and transform that energy into something worthwhile.

I'd love to tell you that once I'd had a couple of these deep, metaphysical revelations, life was smooth sailing from then on. If my life were a movie, this would be where the director would yell, "Cut," the music would swell to a crescendo, and the credits would roll. You'd be left to imagine me as an ever more slender, successful painter. I wish real life were that tidy.

After the paintings were hanging in the gallery and that immediate focus was gone, I found myself sliding back into my old pastimes: watching TV, reading books, and trying not to overeat. Wait a minute. Trying not to overeat? After all, my stomach could only hold half a cup of food at a time. I wasn't having cravings exactly, not like before. At first I didn't really know what was going on.

One night I tried to just sit with those feelings and figure them out, because they weren't going away. I was scared, I was lonely, and for some reason I couldn't get myself to start another painting, but I knew that I needed to do something different and do it now, before the demons had their claws into me so deep I'd never break free. So I went to one of my twelve-step meetings, listened to everyone for an hour, and felt a little better. But not much. As I looked at a couple sitting in the back of the meeting, playing with their toddler, I realized what was bothering me.

Sometimes my deep longing for a family, coupled with the reality of being alone, is so strong I just don't know how to handle it. When the meeting was over I got back onto the highway in a kind of sad trance. Now that it was just me and I didn't have to keep up the façade, I began to cry.

It's never a good idea to cry while driving, as anyone knows. It's dangerous. I could see myself on the front page of the *Maui News:* "Divorcée drowns in own tears while driving, causing seven-car pileup." So I pulled off the road and into a parking lot.

And there, right in front of me, was a grocery store. I stopped crying. I went in and wandered around, ending up in the check-out line with sugar-free ice cream and reduced-fat chips, feeling vaguely guilty like I used to, when I'd been the real fat lady buying the real ice cream.

As I got in the car with my pile of munchies, I was conscious of suddenly feeling much better, like now I could make it through another night alone. I went home and spent the rest of the evening watching mindless TV and nibbling on the snacks I'd bought.

I knew I could have journaled about it, or prayed, or called a friend. But in that moment all I could feel was the hurt, as well as the longing to have a family of my own, to have love and to belong, like everyone else seemed to. What was I supposed to do with these gut-wrenching feelings? That night, the answer was easy and, sadly, all too familiar—eat something.

After my third sugar-free treat, it was nearly 11 P.M., and I decided I needed to tally up my food for the day. I collected paper, pen, and calorie-counting book. Total: 1,350 calories. Actually, not too bad as far as the numbers go.

But what about my failure to stand firm in the face of that storm of feelings—what number could I put on that? Now I began to understand what the eating disorder experts had been saying for years, about how we turn our real problems into pseudo-problems around dieting and weight, because those issues at least *seem* manageable. It was as if I thought I could take all my loneliness and confusion and reduce those feelings into a set of numbers and thus make them more tangible, more solvable.

I can still lose weight on 1,350 calories per day. But I can't recapture the years I lost, or create a family out of thin air. I can't make Eric come back to me. I can have weight loss surgery, drop seventy pounds, and get lots of compliments and praise—but I can't seem to stop wanting this man who is too scared to try again.

I look at the girl in the mirror—the one I so wanted to be—and my friends tell me I'm there now. But inside my head and heart, I'm only just beginning. My body looks a lot better, and physically I feel a lot better—but inside I still feel fat, ashamed, and sad.

Because if I were really so much better, wouldn't Eric want to come back?

People feed you the fantasy that says when you lose the weight, everything will be better. When you lose the weight, your knight on a white horse will show up and carry you off into the sunset, and you'll live happily ever after.

Well, don't believe it. Lose the weight for your health, to feel better inside and out. Lose the weight for your heart and spirit, to free you up to get out there and enjoy life. But don't hold your breath waiting for your knight to show up. Show up for yourself!

Some Methods to Retrain Your Brain
◎

Remember, the old "diet" mentality has got to go! Replace it with small changes that add up to a lifestyle shift, not just a diet. The old "sin vs. virtue" or "bad vs. good" mindset has got to go, too. You know the script: "I was so *bad*, I ate a brownie last night, but today I'll be *good*, I'll only eat lettuce." You are already good, so stop talking about food choices as though you've committed a sin. You haven't.

You are always good enough, just the way you are.

ASSIGNMENT: Replacing Negative Programming with Healthy Affirmations

The table that starts on the next page, "Learning to Honor My Body," lists some negative thoughts commonly reported by people dealing with food and body issues. It also lists some positive affirmations to replace them with. Consider which of the negative messages listed in the table you've thought or said to yourself, and resolve to replace them with healthier alternatives.

It may take some perseverance and mental focus to uncover negative thoughts. They can be so subtle and automatic that sometimes we don't even know they're there. We know we feel bad, but we don't really know why. Often, when you find yourself feeling in despair, discouraged, irritable, or anxious, if you pay attention you can trace those unpleasant emotions back to your negative thoughts. Once you've done that, take a moment to recognize and experience the feeling (affirmations are *not* about avoiding your emotions), and then begin repeating a positive affirmation to yourself.

Use affirmations that are believable to you. Say them aloud or silently, write them down ten times in a row—do whatever you can to incorporate them into your thinking, and get rid of those old negative messages! When you start taking charge of the thoughts parading through your mind, rather than being at their whim, you may be surprised by how much more empowered and content you feel. (I discuss affirmations in more depth in Chapter 9.)

Learning to Honor My Body

Old, negative thoughts	New, positive affirmations
My body isn't good enough (pretty enough, good-looking enough).	My body is my friend and companion throughout my whole life.
I have to battle against my body (or against my food cravings) to lose weight. Sometimes I feel like my body is my enemy.	My body is speaking to me all the time, trying its best to work with me, not against me. I will listen to its voice.
I don't like my body, and neither does anyone else, so I'll just ignore it, stuff it, or punish it with starving/bingeing.	I can't hate my body and love myself at the same time. I choose to love my body as it is right here and now.
If I really let myself go, I'd lose control completely, eat everything in sight, and become a big fat balloon.	If I really let myself go, I'd release all the feelings that get pushed down by food, and then I'd be free to move on.
I hate my _____ (thighs, belly, skin, etc.).	I choose to love my body as it is right here and now.
Food is my best, most reliable comfort source.	With loving practice, I'm learning to enjoy healthier comforts.
I don't want to live on a diet for the rest of my life—it's too overwhelming, and it's no fun!	I don't have to diet! I can still enjoy food, making small changes at my own pace. I can also have fun enjoying new things.
I've always failed before, so why try? I get disgusted, then stress my body with more overeating till I'm sick of that, too!	In the past, I was too hard on myself, trying to change 100 percent overnight. Now I **love** myself into healthier living!
My body is just a prop to carry my head around. It isn't really **me**.	My body is an important part of who I am, every day of my life. My body and I can work together in a loving relationship.

Old, negative thoughts	New, positive affirmations
Only youthful, lean bodies look good or desirable. I judge myself and others if we don't measure up to the highest standards.	All bodies have their own unique beauty, like works of art. I can practice loving acceptance of all our many body types.
Fat people are lazy, sloppy, and gross. Fat prejudice is okay with me.	Being in a larger body doesn't mean anything bad about a person. I can be a voice for change, for body acceptance.
Because I don't look "good," I isolate myself.	I deserve to get out there and enjoy all the good things in life!
When I lose weight I'll _____ (get the job, find the great relationship, etc.).	I'm going for the things I want today, instead of waiting.
When I overeat, I like myself even less.	Each self-loving choice I make helps me break that old cycle. Right now, I am choosing to love myself into better health.
Negative self-scolding has not helped me become healthier.	I am loving myself into a healthy body, mind, heart, and spirit right now.
What are some negative thoughts you might have about your body or your eating that aren't on this list? Write them in your journal.	Then create positive affirmations that are good opposites to your old negative programming. Write them, say them, believe them!

ASSIGNMENT: Examining Body Prejudice

1. Spend an evening in front of the TV (did you ever think I'd recommend such a thing?) and notice the people who appear in the shows, especially in the commercials. How many are slender? How many are overweight, and, if they are, how are they portrayed? As objects of humor or ridicule? Write down how many images or ads promote our society's obsession with thinness versus how many promote a more liberal acceptance of a variety of body types. Two hours' worth of TV should provide you with plenty of "food for thought." Write any other

thoughts about what you saw, and your feelings about it, in your journal.

2. Go to your local mall, one with a bookstore in it, and plan to hang out for an hour or two. Take your journal with you. First, go into the bookstore and flip through some art books that show body paintings from ancient times to the present, especially those portraying the nude female form. Pay special attention to the wide variety of body types and sizes seen as beautiful, like the nudes found in Medieval art, Italian Renaissance art, and paintings by Rubens, Titian, Renoir, Manet, and Gauguin. Can you open your mind and let go of our modern "fat prejudice" enough to see beauty in these images?

3. Next, with your journal, go to a bench or café in the mall and watch the people go by. Imagine each one as the central figure in one of those paintings (I'll leave it up to you as to whether you imagine them with or without their clothes). The point is to try to imagine them as beautiful in their own way, in an artistic sense, whatever their body size. See if this practice makes an impact on your views of beauty or body image in general. Write about any reactions you have.

4. Returning to the "Learning to Honor My Body" exercise, pick one or more of the positive affirmations that feel good to you, and write it or them down on slips of paper. Post them in places where you'll see them, like in your car or on your bathroom mirror. When you see them, say them aloud with heartfelt intent. An even better method is to make a recording of the affirmations in your own voice with some soothing music in the background, and listen to it often (for more on how to do this, see Chapter 9). If privacy is a concern while listening to your recording, you can use headphones or listen to it in the car.

ASSIGNMENT: Visualizing Your Inner "Thin Person"

Let's return to the assignment you completed near the end of Chapter 1, "How I'm Limited Because of My Weight." This time we are going to revisit your answers and use them to create a "mental movie" (also called a visualization) of the fabulous life that can be lived by that wonderful "thin person"—you!

Using your answers from that assignment for ideas and as inspiration, write a paragraph or more about the ideal life of the "thin" you (let's use the term "healthy" instead, shall we?)—the healthy, strong, vital you, who accepts no limitations because of body size. What are you wearing, feeling, and doing? Include as much detail as you can.

Next, step into the movie yourself. Feel and see the scene as clearly as you can. Spend a few minutes there. Tell yourself, "I am living my best life, right now!" Visualize your ideal scene a few times a week.

Now watch as the visualization becomes reality!

Making It
Work
in the Real World

Dear God,

> *Thank You for this day.*
> *So far today, I haven't hurt anybody.*
> *I've been cheerful and kind in all my actions.*
> *I haven't lied, cheated,*
> *Or even had an unkind thought.*
> *But in a minute, God, the alarm will go off*
> *And I'll have to get out of bed.*
> *After that, I'll probably need Your help.*

— Anonymous

It's easy to live well on paper, to think the right thoughts and agree to fully express our feelings. It's easy, when we are by ourselves, to stand firm in our motivation to treat our bodies and ourselves in a healthier way. But all this is put to the test the minute we come into contact with other people! Relationships with our friends, families, or coworkers can comfort us, challenge us, and stimulate us to ever-deeper growth. Unless you're a monk dwelling alone on a mountaintop, your relationships have probably affected the way you eat.

A common pattern I've found among those of us who struggle with food and body issues is a tendency toward codependency. What is codependency? It is a way of relating to others in which we give generously of ourselves while often getting little in return. It is a pattern in which we sometimes end up neglecting our own needs in order to help others meet their financial and emotional needs or other obligations. With only good intentions, we "help" until we are tired and drained, sometimes to the point of exhaustion. And since the people we're helping often aren't able or willing to reciprocate, our own needs get left hanging. So what do we do? We eat. We fill our emotional or spiritual void with food.

◎ Carol's Story

Carol is a friendly fifty-five-year-old woman who loves to have her friends over, and she believes in always maintaining an open-door policy at home. One of her friends, Tracy, is a single mom who has trouble managing her finances. On several occasions Tracy borrowed money from Carol with the promise that she'd pay it back the minute her next check came.

But weeks would pass, and instead of paying Carol back, Tracy asked to borrow more money. When Carol asked her why she hadn't paid back the previous amount, Tracy became tearful and said that her children needed food and clothes, never answering Carol's question about why she hadn't paid her back. This happened several

(cont'd.)

times, and Carol's resentment began to grow. She said, "Of course I wanted her and her kids to be okay, but I'm not rich myself, and my husband was starting to complain about it. I didn't know which way to turn. Between the two of them, I'd get so frustrated that I'd end up eating way more than I should have."

As Carol began to learn about the connection between her eating and codependency, she realized she would need to set some boundaries. "I knew I was going to have to stop being the open wallet for Tracy," she said, "but I was scared to say no. I felt so guilty, like I was being selfish, a bad person. But it had to stop."

At first, when she told Tracy that she would no longer be able to lend her money, Tracy cried and wondered out loud how she was ever going to pay for her children's school clothes. "I felt bad, but I stood my ground," Carol remembered. "After I told Tracy I couldn't lend her money anymore, she sulked at me whenever she came by to visit. She asked for money on a few more occasions, but when I kept to my word, a funny thing happened. She stopped calling or coming over, and after a few weeks, she disappeared altogether. I was hurt, because I realized that she must have been just a fair-weather friend to begin with.

"But one good thing that did come out of all this—besides more money of my own—was that I've become a lot more careful about the kind of person I let into my life. If they can't give as well as take, I don't have time for them. I respect myself more today. That's not to say I've stopped giving, but now, the people I give to care about me enough to give back."

Pulling the Plug on the Energy Vampires

One important way we can identify which relationships are giving us support and which are causing us stress is by taking a hard look at our patterns of give and take within those relationships. Ideally, there will be a flow, a balance between what we offer and what we receive. It doesn't have to be tit for tat, but in a general sense we will feel like we are appreciated, that our time and energies are respected. We don't even have to give the exact same kinds of things; it's more about honoring the spirit of sharing in a relationship. My friend Trisha and I go for walks several times a week, and we've worked out a system. I hate to carry anything when I'm walking, and she hates to drive. So I'll usually drive, and she will carry the water. We are both happy with the result.

Give and take is obvious even in conversations. Have you ever known someone who, when you say, "Hi, how are you?" talks for the next half hour without taking a breath? And when you manage to finally escape you feel drained, have a headache, and make a mental note to avoid that person the next time you see them?

That, my friends, is an energy vampire. An energy vampire is someone who sucks you dry, who drains out all your vital energy, either by ceaselessly going on about themselves or by being so needy that you feel like no matter how much you give to them you're just spitting into the ocean, because they always need more.

How and why do we get caught up in the drama of a relationship with an energy vampire? Usually it's with the best of intentions. We feel sorry for someone in pain and feel good about trying to help them. And if this were a healthy, give-and-take kind of relationship, it would be normal to help each other through the rough times. The trouble is, with an energy vampire, the relationship is out of balance. It's all about them. You end up doing most of the giving no matter what the situation.

Wherever possible, I encourage you to give those people the boot. If you are giving too much of your time, energy, or even money—stop. If you feel resentful, irritable, or hurt by their expectations of you—stop. You don't necessarily need to have a big confrontation about how they are taking you for granted; they probably won't see it that way. Instead, get clear on how much of your time and energy you are *truly* willing to give and when, and let go of the rest. If you stand firm in your decisions, if you stop offering the open door, open ear, or open wallet—

most energy vampires will go away voluntarily and find someone else to feed on.

Making Up for Being Fat

◎

Another reason why many of us tend to have trouble in our relationships has to do with how overweight folks are viewed by society. We are not exactly at the top of the social pecking order, and sometimes we will do more than our share of giving to "make up for" our size. Sometimes we will even accept disrespectful or abusive treatment from others, because we think we don't deserve anything better. Society tells us we aren't worth much—that we can't get a better job, lover, or friend—because of our weight. If we believe this, chances are good that we will take the first prospect that comes along, figuring if *they* want *us,* we'd better go for it, because maybe no one else will.

So there we are, hurt and drained by giving too much or accepting too little from our relationships. What do we do when we feel this way? We eat. For comfort, for nurturing, for numbness. Then we may gain still more weight and entrench ourselves even further in this vicious cycle.

◎ Tommy's Story

Tommy, an eighteen-year-old gay college student, was on the waiting list for WLS surgery when he came to our support group. As he introduced himself and explained why he was there, he said, "Between being overweight and gay, I felt like I'd always been hit with a double whammy by society. I've never tried to hide who I am—why should I? Instead, I became the class clown. I made everybody laugh, sometimes with catty little jokes on others, and sometimes on myself. After a really nasty joke at me, when everybody would laugh, I would too—but inside I felt awful. I wanted them to protest—I wanted them to say, 'No, Tommy, don't put yourself down, we love you just the way you are.' But they never said it—they just laughed at my self-deprecating jokes right along with me. I really had no idea how to make it better—after all, I wasn't going to change them. So I'd go home and eat."

Worth

Not long ago, I watched a *Dateline* special on "lookism." This was a show that explored society's prejudice in favor of people who are good-looking and, conversely, against those who are not. To illustrate this phenomenon, the show's producers ran a little experiment. They sent a group of four actors who were pretending to look for work—two very attractive ones and two ordinary-looking ones—out on mock job interviews. All four actors were of a similar age, were dressed in similar clothes, and had nearly identical resumes. They wore hidden cameras to record what happened on their "interviews."

In every case the interviewers were noticeably friendlier to the attractive "applicants," offering more flexible lunch hours, better promotions, and higher salaries. With the plainer ones they left it at, "We'll call you." The pretty ones were given a tour of the office and offered the job right on the spot. This didn't happen just once, or even several times; *it happened at every interview.* Does this surprise you? Or not?

The *Dateline* episode also showed a few other "experiments," including some mock criminal trials with unsuspecting jury members where, again, the only significant difference was in how the "defendants" looked. Disturbingly, the better-looking criminals were given lighter sentences or exonerated altogether. While to a certain extent we might excuse the job interviewers—after all, one can always get another job somewhere else—how can we excuse putting people in prison based on how they look? Or letting dangerous but attractive criminals get off with no punishment?

Years ago, when I received my first prescription for the weight loss pill Phen-Fen, I was given a promotional handout from the company that made the drug. The brochure quoted a survey of college students, all of whom stated that they would prefer "to marry a drug user, a shoplifter, embezzler, or a blind person, before marrying someone who was overweight." This so-called evidence hit me hard. And, along with every dieter I knew, I went right on using the drug—even after the health warnings about it had been issued—until finally a series of drug-related deaths caused it to be recalled completely. Why would we choose to go on taking this drug in spite of its serious health risks? Because, like that college study stated, we were desperate to lose weight, to be deserving of love, to avoid getting stuck out in the cold, rejected in almost every arena of life due to being overweight. That unpleasant college study only confirmed what I had already experienced.

Though most people wouldn't admit to judging someone solely on their looks, many do feel comfortable judging someone's worth based on their weight. I was fat, so I was told by society that I wasn't worthy. It wasn't that anyone was out to get me personally; it's just the way things were, and everybody knew it. Happens all the time. And nobody really questions it.

Until now. Now there is a large group of individuals, namely WLS post-ops, who have experienced both sides of this prejudice within a relatively short time frame. They've felt the hurt of being snubbed as a fat person, and many of them have also experienced its polar opposite, the positive attention one gets from being attractive. We have developed a certain cynicism where beauty is concerned, maybe even a healthy cynicism. This is why I stress developing your insides, your character, and your spirit at least as much as your body. Because your looks, no matter if you're big or small, will change and fade, and in time it will only be your inner beauty that shines through. If you let it! Love and respect yourself, and those things will come back to you.

Please remind yourself that it isn't just outer beauty that confers the power to be loved and treated with respect. It's something more. And this something more is self-worth. It's a belief in your innate value, a belief that you deserve to be respected and to have good things in life. It's a belief that you don't have to put up with bad treatment from anybody for any reason. Whatever your status, whatever you see when you look in the mirror, remember that a large part of how we're treated by others depends on how much we love and respect ourselves!

Recently, my WLS support group discussed this issue of self-worth. It evolved into a conversation about the fact that many of us had made less than optimal life choices, whether in our relationships, our jobs, or other areas. Many of us had been willing to accept less than we're worth because, being fat, we thought it was the best we'd ever get. We took on other's problems and burdens, carrying more than our share of the load because we felt we needed to do more and be more—just to keep pace with normal-sized folks.

One woman said, "In my relationship, even though I pay most of the bills and do most of the household stuff, including all the childcare, I know my boyfriend feels he could 'do better' than me, just because I'm fat." Another lady replied, "Me, too—except for me, it's about my job. I know I'm smart, I'm a good worker, and I'm always there to help my boss when he gets overwhelmed. He always thanks me and tells me I'm such a lifesaver, but my pay is really low and I haven't had a raise in four years. I'm afraid to ask—because of my weight. I'm afraid he'll tell me I'm lucky to have a job at all. What if no one else wanted to hire me because I'm fat?"

At the end of the meeting one woman said, "Maybe that should be our 'food for thought' this week: What do we really believe we're worth?"

ASSIGNMENT: Determining Your CQ (Codependency Quotient)

We've all heard about measuring one's "IQ"—a person's intelligence quotient, generally accepted as a good indicator of your mental intelligence. The following questionnaire offers a way to take a look at your "CQ"—your *codependency quotient* or, in other words, your emotional intelligence.

Score yourself from 0 to 2 on these questions, based on the following scale:

0 = Rarely/Never   1 = Sometimes   2 = Often

1. Do you look for reassurance/approval from others?

2. Do you have trouble seeing your own good points?

3. Do you fear criticism or judgment from others?

4. Do you overcommit yourself?

5. Do you tend to attract people who need help?

6. Do you feel responsible to help when others have a problem?

7. Do you offer advice when you haven't been asked?

8. Do you care for others easily but forget to care for yourself?

9. Do you put your own needs last, feeling it would be selfish to put them first?

10. Do you have trouble with intimate relationships?

11. Do you cling to relationships from a fear of being alone?

12. Do you avoid relationships due to painful past loves?

13. Do you have a hard time asking directly for what you need?

14. Do you feel more comfortable giving than receiving?

15. Will you abandon your routine to help someone else?

16. Do you give generously to others, then feel resentful when they don't give back?

17. Do you keep on giving in spite of evidence that you're being taken advantage of?

18. Do you have a hard time trusting and honoring your feelings? Do you discount your own perceptions?

19. Do you worry over others' problems more than your own?

20. Do you feel most worthwhile when you are helping others?

21. Do you have a hard time saying no when others want something from you?

22. Do you neglect your personal goals, self-care, and friendships when you're with a partner?

Now add up your score. If you scored fifteen or below, you do not appear to have any problems asking for what you need and setting boundaries.

If you scored from sixteen to twenty-two, you do have some of these issues, and you might want to take better care of yourself in your relationships, creating nurturing time for yourself as well as others.

If you scored over twenty-two, congratulations! You are a bona fide codependent, and you share this job description with many others, primarily women, around the world. You would probably benefit from learning to set clearer boundaries, improving your communication skills, and getting rid of the energy vampires in your life.

ASSIGNMENT: Communication Solutions That Work

Looking over your answers to the above questionnaire, pay special attention to the questions that you answered with a two and about which you also said to yourself, "Oh yeah, I do this one *all* the time." Go back and circle at least two answers that you feel strongly about. Then write down a possible solution for each of these issues and practice using it during the coming week. Record the results in your journal.

For example, if you answered a big "yes" to number 21, having a hard time saying no to others, a solution might be to identify one person or situation in your life where this is an issue. Then practice ways to say no that you can live with, like, "I'd really like to help you out, but I'm just not able to. I have to take care of some other commitments." No big explanations are necessary. Your "other commitments" are to your own health and well-being.

Another way to say no is by using our wonderful high-tech telephone system. You can choose to leave a message rather than get into a discussion with someone, especially when you know that he or she will try to push you into doing what you already said no to. You can also use your caller ID or answering machine to screen your calls. You are not responsible for being the sympathetic ear every time one of the energy vampires wants to unleash their drama on you. You are not responsible for listening to guilt trips from those who want to take advantage of you. You *are* responsible for taking better care of yourself so you won't feel frustrated into overeating or into eating to nurture yourself because no one else is there for you.

◎ Mary's Story

Mary, a thirty-three-year-old mother of two, was married to Raoul, a happy-go-lucky South American native. Raoul expected Mary to take care of him the same way his mother had waited on his father, and for the first few years of their marriage Mary had done so. She nurtured her husband and children lovingly, but often felt taken for granted by them.

"When dinner was over and the rest of my family was relaxing in front of the TV, I'd still be in the kitchen cleaning up," she said. "Sometimes it seemed like I'd been in there the whole day, and irritation would start to boil inside me. I felt it wouldn't do any good to ask my husband for help, so why start an argument? Then I'd find myself eating the leftover potatoes or dessert as I 'cleaned up,' and by the time I was finished I'd feel full, content, even numb. I went on that way for years, never fully realizing all the pounds of hurt and frustration I was storing up, until my doctor intervened when I developed diabetes last year."

As she considered the necessary lifestyle changes she needed to make to undergo weight loss surgery, these patterns in her relationship came to a head. "My husband said I didn't need any surgery," she recalled. "He asked why I wanted surgery. Was it so I would be attractive to other men? At first he refused to take care of the kids while I was recovering from surgery, and he put as many obstacles in my way as he could." Eventually, Mary and Raoul received counseling and were able to make some compromises.

She said, "I guess I never gave much thought to the other side of the picture. All I thought about was how good I'd feel if I lost the weight. After surgery, I realized I was going to have to find a whole new way of communicating with my family, a new way of taking care of myself along with taking care of them."

If you are healthy in body, mind, and spirit you can give from a full cup that is spilling over with compassion, strength, and love. If you never take care of yourself because you're too busy doing for others, then you will be giving from an empty cup, and neither you nor the person you are trying to help will benefit. Besides, taking care of yourself can feel really good! Try relaxing in a bubble bath, reading a good book, indulging in a pedicure, going on a walk—whatever you truly enjoy. You and your loved ones will benefit from a more relaxed, healthier you.

Communication and Conflict-Resolution Skills

◎

Sometimes the right thing to do is to deflect a potential drama using the above methods, and sometimes it's better to face things head-on. When the head-on method of conflict resolution is called for, here are some useful skills to keep in mind.

First, ask yourself, "What's my goal in having this talk? Is it to set a boundary, or to make peace with someone, or just to express what I'm feeling right now?" Hopefully your goal isn't only about winning or making someone see things your way. If you can use the guidelines recommended below, you'll probably get a better result. The real "win" occurs when both people go away feeling better about the situation, not worse.

I developed the following handout for use in my classes, and many of my clients have told me they found it useful. Hopefully you will, too.

Take a look at the behaviors listed on the next page. Those in the left-hand column indicate old ways of relating, many of which we've been raised with, and those in the right-hand column present healthier alternatives. How many of the ones in the left column have you engaged in?

Old Ways of Relating and Healthier Alternatives

Old ways of relating	New, healthier ways of relating
Expecting others to change so I'll feel better	Using my new tools to help myself feel better
Blaming others when I'm angry or upset	Owning all my feelings; seeking a healthy solution
Agreeing to things I really don't want to do	Setting boundaries: "Sorry, but I can't help you."
Expecting loved ones to keep me happy	Enjoying my hobbies, goals, friends, personal time
Always worrying about "their" problems	Focusing on my own health first
Stuffing down my feelings with food	Sharing my feelings with supportive people
Making my loved ones the main focus of my life	Having a "full plate" of my own interests
Acting like a victim when there's a problem	Taking 100 percent responsibility for all my feelings
Taking on other people's burdens; feeling overwhelmed	Letting others handle their own problems
Trying to "fix" other people's feelings or actions	Caring and listening without giving advice
Getting comfort in old, destructive ways	Learning to pray, journal, relax, and have fun!
Trying to "get" them to see it my way	Allowing room for another's point of view
Harshly judging myself or others	Accepting myself and others, even if we disagree
Thinking my way is "right"; acting superior or defensive	Being open to another person's point of view
Using any means to get my way; fighting dirty	Speaking my truth in a kind, honest manner

If any of the statements on the left ring true for you, consider trying some of the alternatives. If any of your words or actions may have caused harm to another person, make your apology as sincere as possible. If no apology is required but you still have something you need to communicate, use the following method.

A Sandwich You Can Still Have

Here is another tried-and-true method for communicating your way through a conflict with the least possible stress. This is called the "sandwich method." It's not manipulation, but it is a formula for speaking your truth in such a way that the other person can take it in easily without getting defensive.

Here's how it goes: The sandwich is made of two slices of bread and one piece of meat. The first piece of "bread" is finding something positive to say about your connection with the other person, something you appreciate about them. It need only be a few sentences, but it should be sincere. People can generally tell if you're just "blowing smoke."

Next comes the "meat." This is the not-so-positive thing that you really need to tell them. Do it briefly, using the communication skills listed in the right-hand column of the chart presented above.

Last comes your second slice of "bread," which is to summarize the situation, state your hope that it can be worked out in a good way, and add one or two more appreciative comments about the other person. All of this "sandwich" method can be done in under five minutes, and it really works better if you keep it as brief as possible. In other words, be sincere, be brief, be done.

At one time I had a roommate whom I wanted to ask to move out. I knew she enjoyed living at my house, and I was really worried about how she would take it when I told her she had to leave, especially considering that, after I told her, we would still be living together until she found a new place. So I used the sandwich method.

I said, "Laurie, I want to thank you for having been such a good roommate over the past year. You always paid your rent on time, and I really appreciate how you helped out around the house." (That was the first slice of bread.) "So I'm truly sorry to have to inconvenience you, but the time has come for me to make a change. I need to have the house to myself. I realize it's a hassle to move, and I'm sorry about that. Please feel free to use me as a reference, and take the full thirty days to find a place you like." (That was the meat.) "Laurie, I just want you to know that you have been a really great tenant, and thank you again for everything. If there's something I can do to help you through this change over the next month, I'd be happy to do it." (That was the second slice of bread.)

After all my worries over what her reaction would be, she was fine, and she actually thanked me for being so nice about it.

How to Navigate Holidays, Parties, and the Dreaded Potluck

◎

Not all of our social interactions have to do with conflict or setting boundaries. Some of them can actually be fun! And when we're having a good time, who wants to stick to a food plan? When all those goodies are spread out on the buffet table, who wants to be the party pooper when everyone else is ooohing and aaahing over the gourmet chocolate cake?

There *are* ways to navigate through these situations without feeling deprived and without eating things you'll regret later. There are ways to enjoy the party, enjoy your food, and leave feeling good about your choices. Here are some tips for how to accomplish this:

- One hour prior to the party, take 1,000 mg of the amino acid L-glutamine and 1,000 mg of DLPA (assuming you've tried these supplements and found them helpful).
- Eat a healthy meal before you go to the party.

- Choose to make your nurturing "food" the time you spend with friends enjoying their company rather than the food on the table.

- Make your own potluck dish or two—something you will enjoy eating (I usually make chili or a stir-fry for a main dish and a fruit salad for a dessert).

- Don't hang out near the food.

- Have at least one support person at the party who knows what your food boundaries are.

This is a time when being really clear about your boundaries around food is vital. For example, I try to steer clear of wheat or sugar products. In this way, if I'm looking at a buffet table, it's pretty easy to figure out what I can and can't eat.

I'm not saying it will be easy, and sometimes, if I'm struggling with cravings, I may either choose not to go to the party or I'll go just long enough to "show face"—meaning I make an appearance out of courtesy to the host—and avoid staying very long.

During the holiday season I plan ahead. I make roast turkey with fresh herbs and a wheat-free stuffing, as well as sugar-free pumpkin custard, sugar-free cheesecake, and sugar-free cranberry sauce with apples and raisins. I make these delectable dishes not just for the parties but also for myself so I won't feel deprived.

Recently I attended an elegant catered wedding held at a beach estate here on Maui. Because there are so many four- and five-star resorts in Hawaii, "catered" usually means you're getting one of those fabulous hotel chefs on their day off, and such was the case here. I was able to pick and choose at the brunch buffet, and I didn't feel deprived because all the food was wonderful, even though I passed over the handmade pastries, croissants, and muffins.

After the meal, the bride stood up and announced that all of the guests would be getting not one but *two* individually handcrafted desserts. "Uh-oh," I thought.

As the waiters in their white coats came around with these lovely, artistic, sugary, sculpted treats held high (including cheesecake, my favorite), I already had several of my usual food boundaries in place. Four people at the table, good friends of mine, knew about my surgery and my weight loss, and since I make no secret of the "no-wheat, no-sugar" food plan, they knew about that, too. I got up before the dessert arrived and fixed myself another plate of fruit and sushi, knowing I probably wouldn't eat it all, but wanting to have it in front of me.

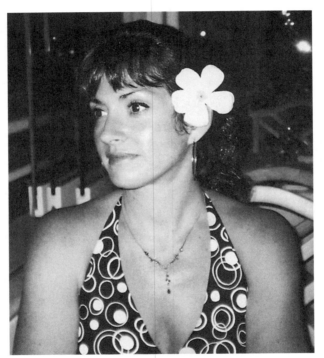

Brunch at the Grand Wailea Resort

Sitting on one side of me was my friend Margaret, and as she dove into her dessert we joked about how many calories were in those beautiful confections. On my other side was a woman I'd just met, who said, "You're not eating the dessert? How can you resist? It's a special day, after all." I wasn't offended. God knows how many hundreds of times I would have said the same thing. I replied, "The thing is, if I eat that, then the sugar demons will get me, and I'll be up at three in the morning driving to the store for Häagen-Dazs!" We had a good laugh and went back to eating our respective meals.

I'm sure she thought I was kidding about the Häagen-Dazs. But you, dear reader, know better, don't you? Food cravings ran my life for over thirty years, and although the dessert did look wonderful, you can keep it.

I prefer my freedom.

Soul Food
The Importance
of Spiritual Nourishment

*When your
spirit feels full,
you do too*

I don't want to turn anybody off when I talk about the importance of having a spiritual connection. I'm not here to convert you to religion—only to offer one more set of tools for one more important area of our lives.

Simply put, a spiritual connection helps us define our place in the world, what we're put here for, and, maybe, what to look forward to when we leave. When we have a sense of meaning and of who we are, why we're here, and what we're meant to do, we feel more centered, focused, and at peace. Having a spiritual foundation can also offer us a sense of hope for the future and a sense of personal power, backed up by the greater power of God, Spirit, or whatever we choose to call It. The Taoists call God "the Great Mystery." I like that.

For many of us, our spiritual or moral guideposts have been replaced by the daytimer, the cell phone, and the clock. As children we heard sayings like, "Do onto others as you would have them do unto you," and "Take time to smell the roses," but the deeper meaning behind those ideas was lost as we grew up and became focused on our careers or other goals. Some of us went to church and were either inspired or disillusioned by what we found there.

Still, the search for meaning in our lives never really went away; it just went underground. We weren't sure how to satisfy it, but we kept trying. There was always someone who claimed to have the answer and was ready to sell us their brand of contentment—for a price. We listened, and we fed that restless, lonely place inside us with the latest clothes, car, or gadget, and we felt satisfied, for a while.

But sooner or later the dissatisfied feeling came back—and the search began again.

For some of us, the restlessness could be soothed by eating something. Food did a pretty good job in the short-term. It made us feel full, satisfied, even numb. But like every other "fix," it was only temporary, and pretty soon we needed something more.

Have you ever found yourself standing in front of an open refrigerator for the third time in an hour, even though you're not really hungry and don't really know what it is you're looking for? Sometimes you're looking for a way to cope with uncomfortable feelings, and sometimes it could be your body trying to talk to you about a lack of nutrients.

Sometimes it isn't any of those things, yet that feeling of wanting *something* is still there. Even though your nutritional intake was fine that day, and you're not upset about anything, still there's this restless feeling seems to have come out of nowhere. Sometimes it is a spiritual hunger, and the only food that will truly satisfy it is soul food.

Many of us thought that the search would end if we just got control over our weight. We believed the fairy tale that promised, "If you lose those extra pounds, you'll be attractive and sought after. You'll feel great about yourself, and everyone will love you."

Putting our faith in that lie has doomed many of us to hopelessness, because we *haven't* lost the extra pounds. We kept waiting—to get the great job or the great relationship—until we were slender. While we waited, we lived in a fantasy world about what would happen once we were thin. While we fantasized, we procrastinated about taking any action toward those goals, and we ate. Time passed, sometimes many years, as we struggled to succeed with our weight, our self-esteem, and our choices.

The diet industry has never really addressed the reasons why we don't stick to their programs. They ignore our struggles or tell us it's our own fault, then they keep offering us another diet. Desperate to live the fairy tale, again and again we go for the proverbial carrot dangling in front of the donkey.

The worst thing about a really good lie is that parts of it are true. It is true that if you are obese and you lose weight you will probably have more opportunities in work and love than you did before. It is true that you may feel more confident as you make better choices about food, and you may carry that confidence into the rest of your life.

It is *not* true, however, that having a better-looking body is a magic wand that will instantly transform the rest of your life. It may make you feel better when you're buying clothes or you're on a date, but it will not give you peace. It won't provide true contentment. How many times have we seen the eighteen-year-old beauty whom we'd kill to look like—yet even she is depressed about the size of her thighs? For her, as for all of us, the answer lies not in another diet, but in developing our heart, mind, and spirit along with our bodies. These are the real keys to feeling good about who you are.

Accepting Where You Are While on the Way to Where You're Going

The most important spiritual attitude I can recommend for gastric by-pass patients, whether pre- or post-op, is to love yourself however you are right now, and to trust that your current circumstances are part of a divine plan, even if it doesn't seem like that's the case. I see so many preoperative patients who are impatient for the surgery, and once they've had it they are impatient for the weight to come off. You may not believe it right now, but living by a healthy nutritional plan and simply taking good care of yourself day to day can give you a feeling of happy self-confidence *regardless of your weight.*

In our "pull-yourself-up-by-the-bootstraps," self-help–obsessed culture, we've been trained to believe that we can accomplish anything or fix any problem if we just put our minds to it. Our society does not support the idea that there are some things we are unable to conquer by willpower alone. The concept of powerlessness—and especially that there's *value* in powerlessness—is difficult for most people to understand.

Accepting our powerlessness over food and body issues means we give up fighting a useless battle and surrender to the truth. "Surrender" here means accepting that some things are bigger than we are and that no matter how hard we try, we cannot surmount them just through the use of our own willpower. It also means that once we leave off fighting, we start putting our energies into the battles we *can* win instead of struggling with the ones we can't.

When it comes to powerlessness over food, we face a battle that has been made doubly hard by the diet industry's insistence that if we can't get a grip on our eating, we are bad, lazy, weak, shameful people. We buy into these notions and end up feeling bad about ourselves, which, ironically, makes us want to eat!

A vicious circle gets set into motion. It starts when we feel some form of stress or discomfort. We begin to crave a yummy treat to help us feel better, but we tell ourselves, "Oh no, I really shouldn't." Our mind bounces back and forth like a tennis ball between "Just go ahead and have it; you know you really want it," and "But I really want to get a handle on my weight," and "Yeah, but just this once won't hurt." On and on it goes, until we give in and eat. Then we feel guilty and promise to "be good" next time. Fueled by guilt, we stick to our plan for an hour or a day or a week—until something else happens. Maybe it's something painful, or maybe it's a celebration. Maybe we can't put a finger on exactly what it is, but something triggers us into overeating, and the cycle begins again.

That cycle was a daily struggle in my life for many years, until I accepted that I was powerless over certain things and certain foods. I kept trying to act like a "normal" person when it came to my eating. It certainly seemed like I *ought* to be able to do that. I judged myself harshly as I compared myself with people who don't have trouble following a diet (usually people who don't have much of a weight problem to begin with).

Acknowledging powerlessness is nothing to be ashamed of. A client of mine, Carrie, a twenty-five-year-old surfer, struggled with sugar binges, then beat herself up because she couldn't have just a little without ending up eating a lot. I used her favorite activity to make a point about powerlessness. I said, "The ocean is bigger than you, right?"

"Yeah, of course the ocean is bigger than me," she replied, looking at me like I was nuts.

"And you know you should never turn your back on the waves, because a big one could knock you off your board, right?"

"I try to be careful. I have a good time, but I always respect the water."

"Well, do you think that knowing that the ocean is bigger than you makes you weak? You're a good surfer, right? You've been out there for, what, the past ten years? How come someone as experienced as you still has to watch out for the waves?"

She laughed and said, "Because you never know when the next big one is going to hit, and you can either ride it or it's gonna ride you!"

"So knowing and respecting the fact that the ocean is more powerful than you actually makes you a better surfer?"

"Definitely," she nodded.

"So, what if knowing you were powerless over sugar could help you respect it enough to just stay away from it altogether?"

She was quiet as she mulled this over, then replied, "I guess if I treated my sugar addiction the same way I treat the ocean, then I'd pay a lot more attention to it, and give its power a lot more respect than I do now."

I smiled and replied, "Because if you don't ride it, it's gonna ride you!" We laughed, but at the same time we were acknowledging the seriousness of her problem.

If we accept the idea of powerlessness, are we stuck being weak, pitiful creatures who are doomed to be fat? Thankfully, no. We can learn to utilize another form of power, one that really works, in the form of spiritual support. We can discover the answers we never found in the refrigerator, no matter how many times we opened it!

What do I mean by "spiritual support"? It can come from a belief in God, or from a belief in nature, or even by looking to a mentor who has already achieved the kind of success we seek. We can use any of these resources as a guide and an inspiration. We can also find or create a safe place to go to when we need to recharge our spirit.

The tools of prayer, meditation, and creating a sacred space are vitally important because learning to get your soul's nourishment from its proper source, instead of from the refrigerator, is vital to your long-term success after surgery. Whatever your spiritual orientation, or even if you don't have one, take heart. There are many ways to develop a side of yourself that will help you feel more positive, serene, and focused. And chances are, if you feel spiritually "full," you won't be tempted to overeat!

Stepping Out in Faith

Like every other gastric bypass patient, you'll eventually face the question of what to do when your appetite returns, your new tummy can hold much more food, and—surprise!—you can eat the same way you did before the surgery. At this point, more than ever, you must introduce some new tools into your life and really make use of them.

In my sixth month after surgery I found myself again "hitting bottom" with my eating. My weight loss had stalled for several weeks. I knew I was floundering and that I needed help. But how could I become the kind of person I'd never been? How could I transform myself from an obese foodaholic into someone who was healthy in body, mind, and spirit—and who could stay that way for longer than a week or two? Was it even possible for someone like me to become "normal"?

I knew that only a spiritual solution could lift me out of thirty years of self-destructive behavior patterns. So I recalled an earlier period in my life, a few years after I'd gotten clean and sober, when I hit bottom with a love relationship and reached out to God, using prayer and meditation for solace.

In doing so, I got much more than I bargained for.

In my early days of being clean and sober, I ate enough sweets for a bakery convention, smoked cigarettes like they were going out of style, and engaged in high drama with my sober but equally dysfunctional boyfriend, Joe the biker. Slowly it dawned on me that although I was certainly healthier than I was when I'd been doing speed, drinking tequila, and smoking joints every day, I wasn't really where I wanted to be. I had made a big step on the way to living a healthy life, but I hadn't made it to the top.

By my third year clean and sober, I finally quit smoking cigarettes and promptly gained fifty pounds. Along with the added weight came the predictable changes in how I was treated—by society, by my boyfriend, even by myself. My head hung lower, my emotions were in turmoil, my inner world was dominated by insecurity and fears of abandonment. Joe and I fought more and more often as my weight climbed, and eventually I was on my own again. After three years with Joe I was going through a breakup, but this time I was sober. I resolved not to eat myself into numbness, and I didn't, but it was hard to face the loneliness without any of my old comforts.

Somehow, I knew that the only thing that was going to help me, to *really* help me, was God.

No doubt that word makes some people nervous. They're thinking, oh, brother, here it comes, the religious pitch. But no, that's not where I'm coming from. I don't care what you call it, whether Jesus or Buddha or Goddess or whatever. There was one guy at a twelve-step meeting I attended who said he visualized *his* God as an old black saxophone player named Max. The important thing is making some kind of contact with Spirit, and realizing that a relationship with Spirit, just like a relationship with a person, needs time, effort, and loving attention if it is to grow.

With Joe gone, I'd often wake up with a black depression threatening to overwhelm me. I'd wrestle down my urge to hide at home, get myself up, and go to the beach. Once I felt the crunch of sand under my feet, saw the crystalline sparkle of the sun on the waves, heard the soft hiss of water as it glided up on the shore and around my ankles, my mood lifted.

This was the beginning of my deeper connection with Spirit. I'd walk down the beach day after day, take in the freshness of the morning, and talk to God. I guess you could call it prayer. After several weeks of this daily ritual, I began to feel gently embraced by God as I prayed, as if a wise and powerful guardian were holding me close, protecting me. I still felt sad about my breakup with Joe, but it was as if something had turned down the volume on it.

In its place I began to feel a new kind of peace. New to me, anyway. Looking back, I guess it was the "peace that passes understanding" that so many spiritual disciples have written about through the centuries. And it did "pass understanding" in the sense that none of my outer circumstances had changed at all. I was still alone, I was still severely overweight, I still had no idea where to go from here. Yet I knew, with a deep sense of certainty, that everything was going to be okay.

As I tuned in to the voice of Spirit within me (it's hard to talk about these things without sounding like a cheap new-age guru), I began to feel drawn toward certain ways of living, and drawn away from others. I began to meditate daily. I didn't have any instructions about how to do it, but I tried anyway. I'd turn off the phone, put on some mellow instrumental music (what I call "angel" music), and begin. I'd start by being mindful of my breathing, then visualize a seed slowly growing into a vast tree with each breath. My mind really needed something to keep it focused; otherwise I'd be off in all directions, thinking about the grocery list, or what Joe was doing, or whatever, not exactly spiritual. So the music and the breathing and visualizing the tree all helped me become still inside.

It took time. At first I could only sit for ten minutes or so, then ten became thirty, then sixty. After a month, I was meditating for up to two hours a day, effortlessly going within to the place from which this vast peace emanated. As I experienced it, this inner sanctuary was dark, like being inside a womb or floating through space. It felt like a close embrace, yet at the same time it stretched away into infinity. See? It's not easy to put these experiences into words without sounding like a nut.

But it was real, it was powerful, and it was changing me, slowly and subtly. All the weight I'd gained during my hard times with Joe came off again as if by magic. But, of course, it didn't happen by magic. It happened because I was filling myself up with something more wholesome, a truer nourishment. I drew a kind of sustenance from my meditation, a "daily bread" of loving reassurance from Spirit. Wanting to immerse myself in this way of life, I began to read spiritual books from a variety of cultures and religions.

There's a funny thing about God's will. We agonize and philosophize over what it is, what it isn't, and whether or not we're following it. Wars have been fought and endless debates spun out of the idea that one faction or another is doing "God's will." Since I've yet to see it printed in big letters across the sky like "Surrender Dorothy," I guess the nature of God's will is still open to debate and always will be. But I've discovered a fairly simple answer to the question of what God's will is. It has to do with tuning into a higher frequency, if I dare use that word.

With the idea of frequency comes the ancient spiritual practices of meditation and purification. If my mind and body are at least somewhat clear and free of interference or "static," then I can tune in and hear that higher frequency more clearly. Meditation in particular has helped me to feel inspired and motivated to pursue healthy practices and goals.

Meditation may seem like a vague, otherworldly pursuit better left to priests and monks. How can it be relevant to weight loss, or to following a food plan? Well, there are some things I can't fully explain; as I said, you must try them to understand how and why they work. If you are as desperate as I was, then you will be willing to make the effort. After all, how many crazy diets have we gone on, taking it on "faith" that they would save us from ourselves?

If you already follow a specific religion or spiritual path, you may have some real strengths in this area. Most religions offer guidance in how to pray, and some also have certain practices to help clear your mind through meditation. If you don't have any background in these practices, or if the whole God/spirituality concept is one you don't feel comfortable with, don't worry. No one is trying to convert you. We can still look at some simple, straightforward methods you can use to help you feel more grounded, serene, and hopeful.

Consider it this way: Any time I eat for reasons other than nutrition (which used to be most of the time), it's usually due to my being upset in some way—angry, lonely, overwhelmed, or exhausted. When I pray and meditate, I find a sense of peace that lowers the volume on these other emotions, and I'm less likely to overeat. The "daily drama" doesn't seem quite as big or important, and instead of my just reacting to things, I feel like I have a little breathing room—to take a step back, consider my options, and respond in a healthier manner.

Some benefits you can receive from prayer and meditation are—

○ a clearer mind, one that is less scattered or distracted

○ a positive attitude; being less fearful or negative in your outlook

○ an improved ability to focus your mind and energy on your goals

○ a heightened sense of intuition

○ an ability to be more "present" in every moment

○ less fear, more peace

○ less irritability, more patience

○ a sense that everything will be okay; less worry

○ a more loving acceptance of yourself and others

Do these qualities sound like they're worth having? They are what I call the "evidence," because when I meditate regularly, I can see and feel them become more prominent in me. And when I look at people whom I admire, who have a way about them that is loving, peaceful, and grounded, I usually discover that they, too, follow a regular practice of prayer and mediation.

ASSIGNMENT: Building Your Spiritual Strength

All of the above qualities are available to you if you learn how to use prayer and meditation. That's the good news. The other news is that it doesn't happen overnight. In fact, the first few times you try meditating you may feel like it's a waste of time. You'll have to follow the practice for at least a little while to see the benefits. In this respect, it's a lot like going to the gym for a workout. If I go to the gym once in a while, or even just once a week, all I get is sore. Being sore doesn't exactly make me want to go back and do it again, so I may stop altogether. However, if I commit (there's that word again) to going to the gym at least three days a week, my muscles will start to build, I'll stop being sore, and I'll start to see results: a firmer, more toned body.

The same thing goes for meditation. At first, when you try to sit still, breathe deeply, and quiet your mind, you'll probably feel squirmy and distracted. Every time you try to focus on your breathing, or on an image like a candle or a tree, within seconds you'll be thinking about the laundry list, or what you're going to have for dinner, etc. You'll think, "Geez! I never realized it would be this hard to just get my mind to *shut up!* It's impossible!"

It's not impossible. It just takes practice. And like going to the gym, you will see real results only with consistent practice several times a week. If you have time to meditate daily or every other day, great. If you do it less than three times a week, all you'll probably get is frustrated.

Here's a method to try:

- o Set aside ten to thirty minutes of undisturbed time. "Undisturbed" means you take the phone off the hook, put on some soothing instrumental music to drown out any household noise, and ask the people around you to leave you alone for that period of time. Wear comfortable clothes, light a candle, turn off the lights, and seat yourself in a comfortable position.

- o Use a timer that you don't have to think about, like an egg timer, or the length of a cassette tape or CD. I use a twenty-five-minute cassette of angel music; when it clicks off, I know

I'm done. If I want to keep going, I turn the tape over. Sometimes I use a full-length CD (forty-five minutes). The point is not to have to think about the time.

o   To start, give your mind an activity to focus on, such as one of the following meditations:

Healing golden light meditation: Count to four while you inhale slowly, and then count to six while you exhale slowly. Do this three times to establish a rhythm. Now add the following visualization: Imagine a healing golden light gradually filling every part of your body with each inhalation. With each exhalation, breathe out any tension, stress, or negativity, which you can visualize as a dark mist. Do this for at least ten minutes and you'll find it's as good as a massage or a hot shower for relaxation.

Tree of life: This one is my favorite. It involves visualizing a tiny seed growing into a tree, and watching it grow a little more with each breath. Start by breathing in slowly. As you do so, imagine drawing up powerful creative energy from the Earth's very core, filling up your spine and then your whole being with an orange-gold, energizing light. This is meant to ground you and to provide energy to create the tree. Then, with each exhalation, grow a bit more of your tree. Start by visualizing the seed sprouting, then see a little more of the tree emerging with each breath. It begins as a new green seedling, then develops branches, leaves, and, once the tree is fully grown, flowers and fruit. I usually spend the last few minutes of this meditation visualizing the flowers and leaves of my tree releasing oxygen back into the air. This is a way of completing the circle, giving back the energy I drew from the Earth's core. I always feel both grounded and energized after this particular meditation.

o   Make time to meditate at least three times a week, more often if you can. Write it down in your appointment book if that will help you remember to stick to it.

Another way to honor your spiritual side is to create a sacred space in your home. Some people call it an altar, but it doesn't need to be as formal as that. Many cultures, from

Christian to Buddhist, follow the practice of decorating a designated spot in the home, located in an alcove or on a side table, with candles, flowers, and perhaps photos of loved ones or of a spiritual teacher. Your sacred space could be as big as a whole room or as small as a dinner plate—as long as the elements in it remind you to honor Spirit. You can use your sacred space as a place to pray, especially first thing in the morning or last thing before bedtime. You can use it for meditation, or as a place to go whenever you need to refocus yourself and ask for help from Spirit.

ASSIGNMENT : Making a "Happy Endings" Box or "God" Box

One of the tools my clients have found both fun and useful is making a "God box" or "God can." (Those of you who don't feel comfortable using the "God" word might call it a "Happy Endings" can.) This is a container in which you place written prayers and affirmations. Use it when something is really bothering you and you want to surrender it to the higher workings of the universe (what I call "Spirit"). In my classes we often turn this into a craft project. Each person covers a coffee can or shoebox with pretty fabric or a photo collage and cuts a slit in the top. On slips of paper we write our heartfelt wishes or our problems—our "prayers"—then stick them in the can for Spirit to solve. We say, "If I can't, God 'can'" (that's our little joke). We glue the top onto the can to make sure that, although there is a way to put things *in* the can, there is no easy way to get them back *out*—symbolizing that once we've given our cares to God, we leave them there!

Here's another creative solution I tried.

The Cactus on the Couch

No matter how hard we try or how spiritual we become, old habits always find a way to crop up. If we let them get a foot in the door, they may have the sneaky, yet serious, potential to derail our growth. We can ignore them, we can resist them, or, as this next story illustrates, we can try handling them creatively and with a little humor.

By my sixth month out from surgery, I had lost over fifty pounds. I was able to eat virtually anything I wanted in small quantities, but for the most part I stuck to protein, veggies, and fruits. I still stayed completely away from sugar and most starches. Once in a great while I'd have some sugar-free ice cream or fat-free chips, but, frankly, neither of these was yummy enough to tempt me into any kind of binge. I still had no cravings—at least no physical ones.

But my emotional and psychological cravings were alive and well, darn it. The gobble gremlin's best tactic was to keep me thinking about something else while I wandered around the house with a handful of almonds or an apple. Then when I'd write down my food intake for the day, there were always a few bites of food I couldn't quite remember. My weight was going down again, but slowly.

Then there was my worst foe: a certain corner on the couch, my favorite spot, in fact. It was cozy and close to the TV, and located next to it was a table filled with books and magazines and, usually, food. Healthier food than in the past, but it was still food. However, I could always feel virtuous if I read a self-help book while I nibbled on something.

I realized that even though I'd made a good start, even though I'd had and might still have some setbacks—I had managed to keep moving forward. But the whole point of getting clean and sober, and finally getting off the food, was to be able to fulfill my dreams of being an artist and writer, of being a spiritually centered woman. Of being whole.

Getting rid of an addiction is probably the hardest and most rewarding thing a person can ever do. Unfortunately, it doesn't automatically give us a treasure chest full of goodies. It will clear out some of the obstacles in our lives and free up space for something new to happen. It provides us with a wonderful opportunity to utilize the all gifts we've been given. But it's still up to each of us to do the work.

One night, while sitting in my favorite corner of the couch once again, I asked myself, "So what gifts am I utilizing? Hand-to-mouth coordination?" I felt pulled between the familiar contentment of doing not much and the growing spirit inside me that wanted to create something, or pray, or move my body and breathe. The fragile new buds of this creative spirit needed all the nurturing I could give them—and here I was, letting the demons jump up and down on them while cackling with mischief.

I had to do something.

So I prayed, asking for Spirit to show me what I should do. An unexpected image came into my mind. In response I said, "You've got to be kidding, God." At first, I dismissed the idea, but it kept coming up. (I did mention that my God has a weird sense of humor, right?) After about the third day of repeatedly seeing the same picture in my head, I gave in. "Okay, God, this seems pretty strange to me, but what the heck. I'll try it."

Following my strange inner vision like Moses in the desert, I went to the Kula Hardware and Nursery. They were known to have the best supply of unusual plants in the area, and what I wanted was unusual, at least for Maui. As I entered the nursery, I was enveloped in a cool, fragrant mist. As far as the eye could see, the place was full of lush tropical greenery, elaborate statues, exotic fruit trees, and flowers. One of the salespeople approached me.

"I'm looking for a cactus," I said. "A big one, with long thorns. Do you have anything like that?"

He didn't bat an eye. Instead, he directed me to an area where, true to the store's reputation, they had about thirty different varieties of cacti. I found myself especially interested in the more wicked-looking ones. Some of the best were in really small pots, which they seemed to burst out of, hundreds of little thorns standing at attention on each plant. They were even pretty cheap.

"Maybe I'd better get two," I thought. "After all, the couch does have two corners." I took them home and, just like my inner picture had been guiding me to do, placed each one in a corner of the sofa. Now I literally couldn't sit in my "rut" without getting a bottom full of thorns! For me, the cacti symbolized the perils of allowing myself to become too deeply embedded in comfortable old habits. It may have been extreme, but it worked.

So how can we get ourselves off the couch and moving on to more fulfilling pursuits? Like I did with the cacti, you'll have to take some ideas on faith—that is, you'll just have to give them a try before you see their value. I encourage you to take up meditation or prayer if it suits you, and to create a space and time in your home for peaceful, restorative retreat. I know giving yourself the gift of quiet time can be challenging. We are all busy people with lots of important things to do. Yet if you never replenish your own energy, what do you really have to give to others? Here's a story that may inspire ideas for how to carve out some personal time for yourself.

◎ Terri's Story

My client Terri, a thirty-five-year-old cosmetologist, lived with her large family in a small two-bedroom house. Between taking care of her husband's elderly mother and her niece's twin daughters, and making meals for the family, it wasn't easy for her to find time alone to pray and meditate. I asked her, "Where and when can you have some time to yourself?" She thought about it and replied, "When I'm in the bathroom is just about the only time I get to be alone." So we worked with that.

In the evenings, after work and after her family ate dinner, she would light candles and take a bubble bath, relaxing in the warm, steamy water. While in the tub she would pray, reviewing her day with Spirit and asking to be shown any lessons she needed to learn. She would ask to be forgiven for any mistakes she'd made, and for help becoming a more loving, peaceful person. She'd ask for blessings for those she loved, and especially for those she was having problems with. Finally, after her prayers were complete, she'd get quiet and open her heart in meditation, listening for the voice of Spirit.

At first, what she usually heard were the voices of her kids as they banged on the bathroom door! They wanted to know what the heck she was doing in there, and when she was coming out. They weren't used to Mom taking any time for herself. But, as often happens when we set boundaries, once they got over their initial resistance to change, they began to respect Terri more and to see that she was a person in her own right, with some needs of her own.

Terri herself wasn't even sure if this little "time out" was really worth it. "I felt awkward and selfish at the beginning," she told me, "and my mind kept running on about all the things I needed to get done for the kids, for work, you name it. But as time went on and I kept doing my 'bubble bath retreat' for half an hour each evening, I began to relax and just enjoy the feel of the hot water and the soothing smell of the bubbles. I slowed down and my stress mellowed out. Sometimes I'd pray, and sometimes I'd just breathe deeply and be open to whatever God wanted to show me. I'd see images of art, images from my childhood, unexpected solutions to problems I was having—all kinds of things. It became something really special, just 'me' time."

After a while even her family members began to be protective of her "private time." If the phone rang for Terri she'd hear them say, "Sorry, Mom's busy right now—you'll have to call back later."

Terri said, "When I heard that, I realized my family was beginning to support me, and to help me help myself. It made me all the more motivated to keep up my spiritual work, so I can be the best person I can be, for myself and for them."

That's all any of us can do—make the effort day by day, and listen to the voice of Spirit inside that calls us to be the best we can be. Let's remind ourselves that it's about progress, not perfection, and also that we find our most nourishing soul food in those small moments of contentment along the way.

chapter
eight

Letting Go
of
Old Baggage

*Don't let it
drag you down*

Thus far, we've looked at several possible answers to the question "If I know I really want to lose weight, then *why* do I keep overeating?" To the "civilians" in our society—those who are unafflicted with food or body issues—the issue may seem pointless. But many of us have asked ourselves this seemingly contradictory question over and over again, with increasing desperation as our health conditions, both physical and emotional, grew worse. There is one important topic we have yet to address, and it is crucial to our long-term success. It's hard to talk about, but if we don't, we may end up sabotaging every attempt to reach our goals.

The topic I want to address is that of dealing with old baggage, old trauma, and unhealed wounds stemming from family problems or other early experiences. Even if you've already undergone weight loss surgery, if you're having trouble losing weight or keeping it off, old baggage may be the underlying cause.

Sometimes our feelings about traumatic events were so painful that we just stuffed them down, hoping they'd go away on their own. We'd move on with our lives, perhaps not even realizing that we were covering up a festering wound with food, with other substances or activities, or with "keeping busy." As a result we left a part of ourselves unhealed and hurting. Most therapists and psychologists agree that unhealed parts of ourselves don't go away; they just go underground, creating fears and unhappy beliefs about ourselves and the world. And, sometimes, living life hiding behind these fears and beliefs can hurt us even more than the original trauma did.

◎ Sandy's Story

Sandy is a fifty-two-year-old seamstress and mother of two grown children who attended one of my classes. She was brave enough to reveal that early childhood incest may have been part of the reason why she was having trouble losing weight.

(cont'd.)

She shared, "When I was eleven my grandfather moved in with us. He lived with our family for the next several years, and for all of that time he molested me. He came into my room at night and threatened me with terrible things if anyone ever found out. He told me that if I said anything the police would come and take me away to a foster home. I was terrified. I hated the abuse and hated him, but I didn't know what to do.

"I didn't tell.

"I escaped by getting married to my first husband when I was sixteen. By the time I was twenty I'd had three children and had gained quite a bit of weight, and I've kept the weight on ever since. I often wonder if keeping this weight on me has been a form of protection so no one will look at me or try to hurt me the way my grandfather did."

If you have unresolved hurts in your past, like Sandy did, I encourage you to find a way—a safe, supportive way—to let them out and work through them. We don't have to carry around those old "ghosts" or allow them to continue contaminating our lives. There are counselors, support groups, and many wonderful books that deal with how to heal from childhood trauma. It is possible to work through it and come out on the other side as a stronger person. I know because I did it.

The Fallout from Being Thin

In the summer of 1977, I went on my first big adventure. I had just turned fourteen, and I was traveling three thousand miles away from home by myself. I was going to Maui, Hawaii, to visit a friend of the family. Freedom! Excitement! I couldn't wait!

Teenage girls have a capacity to bend and twist their age depending on the experiences they've had—or missed. A fourteen-year-old girl can look and act much older than she actually is—"fourteen going on thirty"—or she can still be a child, as I was. When I left the mainland to spend the summer on Maui, my body looked like that of a chubby little girl. I was flat, and fat.

Boys were still a mystery to me. Most of the other girls in my class had been going to school dances, dating, and "going steady" for the past year. Some of them had even had sex. I wasn't one of them. There was a clique of girls at school who talked about that stuff, and they'd gained some sort of teenage wisdom about how to deal with boys in this new way. Not me. By the time I arrived on Maui, I'd never had a date, had never even been kissed.

I stayed with a friend of my mom's, Julie, and her family, and I fell in love with them from the beginning. Julie treated me like one of her own kids, with an easygoing familiarity that made me feel at home. She had a garden full of papayas and bananas, and tiny geckos ran up and down the walls day and night. The air smelled of plumeria flowers and the sea.

After taking a compassionate look at me in a bikini, Julie began a clandestine campaign to help me lose weight. It was just a short walk from their house to the beach, so she suggested we go swimming in the ocean—not just playing in the surf like most tourists do, but really getting out beyond the waves and doing the crawl for an hour at a time. At first I was a little frightened, but Julie taught me to understand the cycles of the waves and when it was safe to go into the water.

And so we swam. Boy, did we swim, almost every day. Snorkeling, that seemingly banal tourist sport, opened up a whole new world for me, of beautiful jewel-toned fish and mysterious blue depths. We drank Tiger's Milk drinks, an early precursor of protein drinks, and we kept swimming.

At first I didn't realize it, but my body was changing fast. Inside of a month I went from a pudgy kid to a slender, tanned young woman, with long hair burned golden by the sun and a strong and muscular body from swimming. For the first time in my life I began to feel a measure of self-confidence. Some of it came from the inside, from looking into the mirror and seeing a pretty girl instead of a fat kid, and from feeling the strength and stamina of my new body. Some of it came from the outside, because every time Julie and I went into town, I got noticed. All of a sudden I was being treated differently than ever before. Everyone, it seemed, was suddenly smiling at me and saying hello. Boys my age and older were looking my way, asking my name, even wanting my phone number. When Julie saw that I didn't know how to handle these guys' attention, she would swoop in like a mother hen and tell them to back off. I was relieved but sometimes a little disappointed, especially if it was a cute boy my age!

After I had spent about five weeks on Maui, Julie sent me to stay with her sister Rose in Lahaina, thinking I'd enjoy seeing another part of the island. Rose was a flamboyant forty-two-year-old woman who looked no older than thirty, and she was a member of the hippie culture that was prevalent on Maui at the time. I quickly began to hero-worship Rose. She treated me like an adult and a friend. She talked with me about whatever was happening in her life and let me try on her bikinis. She even let me smoke pot, which I'd already tried back in California. It didn't seem strange, just one more way in which she was allowing me to be an adult. It felt like a magical time, and in some ways it was, with Rose and me sashaying up Front St. in our skimpy bikinis and lacy cover-ups. It was the hippie 1970s on Maui, and anything could happen.

And anything often tried to happen. We ran into a lot of men on our walks, some of whom Rose knew. They treated her with a kind of touchy-feely familiarity, and in the spirit of our new friendship she confided to me that some of them had been her lovers. She seemed to know how to handle men, so their interactions appeared harmless to me. At the time, I didn't realize that a need for "handling" certain men —i.e., for flirting without getting caught up into anything—even existed. But I was about to learn.

One day we went to watch a soccer game that one of Rose's men friends was playing in. As we sat at a picnic table under the trees, two strange men joined us. They wanted to smoke a joint with us, and as we got to smoking and talking, they offered to take us to a beautiful jungle pool about an hour away, ostensibly to go swimming. To my surprise Rose decided we should go with them, even though she'd never met them before. Of course I trusted her judgment.

We got into their van (didn't everyone have a cool hippie van in those days?) and off we went. Eventually we came to the cliffs of Huelo, a wild and beautiful place with incredible pools and waterfalls right out of a fantasy. People had congregated at a house that sat near the cliffs, and soon everyone except Rose and me dropped their clothes to go for a swim. One of the men actually carried Rose, swooning-maiden style, down the steep trail to go swimming.

Somebody broke out a vial of LSD, and nearly everyone took some. I was too scared to try it, but Rose had some. Beer, food, and joints eventually appeared as well. It was turning into quite a party.

The two guys we'd met at the soccer field seemed to want to know all about me. They asked about my home back in California and what grade I was in at school. While we were talking, one of them started giving me a foot massage. The other guy kind of barked at him and told him to leave. Now it was just me and this man, who seemed very gentle and soft-spoken even though he was clearly much older than I was. He suggested we go up to his van for a cigarette. Rose and the rest of the group didn't notice when we left. I'm sure that you, dear reader, can see what's coming, but at the time, I didn't.

Once we got to his van, his manner became much more aggressive. He pushed me down in the back of the van and held me there. "This will be so great for you," he said as he unfastened his pants, "especially since you're a virgin." Did I tell him no? Yes, many times. Did I try to get away? Of course. I was frightened, confused, humiliated—hurt physically and spiritually that night in ways that never fully disappear.

Would he have gone after me if I had still been the fat kid? I doubt it very much.

Several hours later, as the sun was rising, I got away from him when he fell asleep. I went down to the house where Rose was sleeping off the party. I knew she would fix it somehow—that as my friend and the adult in charge of my welfare, she would somehow avenge this nameless injustice. She would protect me. I was crying and shaking, yet at moments I also felt strangely calm. I didn't know what to say about what had happened to me. I don't even remember if I knew to call it rape. But, as I told Rose what had happened, it was surely obvious that I was traumatized and very upset.

Her reaction caught me totally off guard. "Well," she said, looking disgusted, "if you can't handle yourself with men any better than that, I guess I can't take you out with me anymore." She didn't want to hear any more about it. She shook out her hair and applied some lipstick in the mirror. Turning to look at me, she said, "You'd better not tell your mother about this, or I'll never hear the end of it." She looked at me in the same way the pretty girls in my school used to, with disgust and disdain.

Somehow we got through the rest of my visit. My hero-worship of her disappeared, and in its place arose hurt, confusion, and, ultimately, silence. I don't remember much more of the next few weeks. I remember my hands shaking as I tried to hold a teacup. I remember wondering aloud if I were pregnant, and I remember Rose getting angry with me for talking about it. I remember her passing me back to Julie for the rest of my stay, presumably because I couldn't "handle" myself, but more likely because she refused to face the fallout from her own poor judgment and lack of decent guardianship.

As far as I know, Rose said nothing to Julie or to my mother about the incident, and she told me to keep quiet too. Nothing about it was ever mentioned again. At the end of the summer, I flew back to California to begin my freshman year of high school.

By spring of the following year I had regained all the weight I had lost during my wonderful swims with Julie, plus I added thirty more pounds, a pattern that was to plague me for the rest of my life. I had figured out that it was not safe to be pretty. Maybe Rose was right; maybe I just couldn't "handle it."

Overweight and isolated, waddling up and down the halls of my high school, I no longer had to handle anything. None of the other kids wanted to be seen hanging out with a fat girl, and even though I was lonely, it was just…easier. All the boys kept their distance, and that was just fine with me.

I kept quiet about the rape for many years, until I got into recovery and learned that it was possible to heal from such traumas and get on with life in a healthier manner. I did that—I started therapy and did some reading, some writing, some feeling, and some healing. By the time I underwent weight loss surgery, I had no problem standing up for myself when a difficult situation arose—as you'll see in this next journal entry.

Not Safe

◎

This morning I took my dog, Hoku, on a walk up the mountain, along a well-used trail in the pineapple fields. As I'm sitting down to write this, my heart is still pounding, my breath still caught in my throat. I just got off the phone with the Maui Police Department.

I guess I'm calmer now. Calm enough to sit down and write this, even though my hands are still shaking a little.

Here is what happened: We went on our usual hike, up through the pineapple fields like we always do. The country road alongside the field is isolated, but I take my dog to feel safe. When I was deciding eight years ago what kind of puppy to get, I knew I wanted a Rottweiler. I think they're beautiful dogs, and I like the fact that they are protective. In fact, I ultimately decided on the breed because I so enjoy hiking in the woods, and there wasn't always someone around to go with me. With my Rottweiler, I would feel safe. Since then, I've never had any trouble hiking in the forest, not with Hoku by my side.

During the many times I've walked this trail, there were a few incidents when a car would slow down or even stop, the male driver looking over at me from the road as I hiked up the hill. Sometimes it would be two men. They'd look at me, not speaking, not moving. I'd keep them in the corner of my eye, feeling wary, but what could I do? There was no law against stopping and looking. I'd keep walking, but I'd also keep an eye on the car.

But then my dog would pass through one of the open spaces where you could see her from the road, trotting behind me with her happy Rottweiler self, unaware of anything except her enjoyment of the day. And every time she became visible from the road, that car would suddenly start up and drive away. Every time.

I leave it to you to guess those men's intentions, but to me they seemed pretty clear. They wanted to do me some kind of harm, and my dog scared them off.

Maybe you think I should have just stopped walking in those pineapple fields. There were times when I thought so, too. Although it had been more than twenty years since I'd been raped, some things never completely go away. And one of them was the fear I felt whenever a strange man looked at me in a funny way. Still, I refused to let my fear control me. I had the law behind me. I had my Rottweiler beside me. Shouldn't that be enough?

Well, today it wasn't. We were walking up the trail, me with my headphones on as usual, when I saw a man in an old truck driving very slowly up the road alongside me, looking at me. When he saw me watching him, he sped up a little. I picked up a couple of grapefruit-sized rocks and just stood there for a minute, listening. I was behind some tall grass where he couldn't readily see me. I could still hear his truck, so I peered through the grass. Now he had turned around, come back, and pulled over on the shoulder of the road directly across from me. He was just sitting there with his truck idling, staring across the road at me, not speaking.

Now, mind you, there's nothing else around there, no pretty flowers to pick, no lovely view, no homes or mailboxes or anything except the road and the trail. Plus, he'd turned his truck around and parked right next to me. By now, all my internal danger signals were going off. He got out of his truck, looking intently at me through the grass, still not speaking. This was crazy! I wished there was someone to run to, but there wasn't—only the occasional car driving by.

Then he saw Hoku and took a few steps backward. I also made sure he saw the rocks I was holding. He got back into his truck, whipped it around in the middle of the road, and revved the engine. "Thank God he's leaving," I thought.

But he didn't leave. Still looking at me, he revved the engine again and gunned the truck right up and over the embankment between the road and the trail, coming straight at us. The embankment provided enough of an obstacle that he had to go slow. I didn't wait to see where he would go next—I just grabbed Hoku by the collar and ran. We hid in the tall grass a little ways down the trail, me holding the dog's muzzle so she couldn't bark and give us away.

Now he was up on the trail in his truck, driving forward, then back, hunting for me right where I'd been standing. The whole thing seemed so insane, so surreal, that I wasn't as scared as I probably should have been. I was afraid, but I was also really angry. Damn him! I had my dog, I had a massive rock in each hand, and I was going to nail the son of a bitch if I had to. Adrenaline and rage shored me up as I waited to see what he would do next.

He drove back and forth a few more times, but he couldn't see me in the grass, and I wasn't about to jump out and confront him. I was furious and scared, but I wasn't stupid. Who knew if he had a knife or a gun?

"Please, God, please make him go away," I prayed over and over. I waited, holding on to Hoku. I hoped that between the dog, my big rocks, and my readiness to fight back, he would decide I was too much trouble. Finally he drove away, the sound of his engine becoming faint and then disappearing as he sped up the hill.

I waited a while longer to see if he would return. Nothing happened. I got back onto the trail and looked around. The landscape was empty except for Hoku, who was looking up at me and thumping her tail on the path, sending up clouds of red dust. I walked quickly in the direction of my car, which was still a good half mile down the hill. Every time a car came by, I whirled around in a panic—but it was just everyday folks, many of them waving and smiling to me. Just as though some crazy stranger hadn't tried to hurt me. Just as though it were a normal day.

I wanted to scream aloud, not just with fear but with rage. I wanted to bare my teeth like an animal and scream a challenge to that man, to any man who would try to take advantage of a woman as if he had a right to. I was thinking of the women in Africa and the Middle East, and how we act like it's so different here. But a woman here is still not free to go for a walk without fearing for her safety. I almost *wanted* him to come back so I could throw one of those big rocks through his windshield and the other one right at his head.

I hurried to my car and drove home, where I locked the door behind me. I went around the house and locked the rest of the doors and windows. Hoku followed me from room to room, sensing something amiss. I finally sat on the floor and hugged her hard. Then I started to shake. I curled up in a chair and called my friend Lisa.

"You should report it," she insisted.

"But I didn't even get a license plate number or anything, so what could the police do? They'll probably just tell me to stop walking in the pineapple fields," I said.

Lisa said, "Maybe, but whoever that guy was, what if he's doing that kind of thing to a lot of women? Maybe if you just tell them what he looked like and what his truck looked like—at least then they'll have some record of it, in case he tries again with somebody else."

That reasoning got to me. "Okay, I guess I'll call."

But after we hung up, I didn't call. Instead, I sat there and stared at the wall, thinking about all the doors and windows in my house that should really be made more secure, with better locks. I thought about buying another Rottweiler puppy since Hoku isn't getting any younger.

I closed my eyes and sighed, letting out a long breath full of anxiety, fear, and sadness.

I thought about the fourteen-year-old me, who'd lost her virginity through rape. And I thought about being kidnapped in Oakland by two strange men when I was seventeen, and raped again. I thought about how I'd slept with a big butcher knife under my pillow for years afterward, and how I'd gained weight once again to become unattractive. And it worked! During all those years when I was so big, no man had ever threatened me in that way again.

But now I had lost the weight. I had a figure instead of being a big shapeless blob. And here came the threat again. But this time, I wasn't a scared teenager. I was a grown woman, seasoned by twenty years of having to stand up for myself. I wasn't about to back down, or back off, or go hide behind a wall of fat again.

Never again.

"Bring it on, you son of a bitch, " I said, so loud that Hoku jumped to her feet, alarmed. "This is my life, and I'm not going to let you scare me back into hiding."

Almost as an afterthought, I added softly, "And thank you, dear God, for saving me from that guy."

Then I picked up the phone and dialed the police.

Hoku is getting steak tonight.

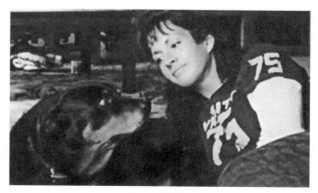

Me and Hoku

How to Heal Old Wounds

Before including any assignment in this book, I tried it on myself first. After doing each of these exercises and experiencing some relief and personal growth as a result, I began using them in my Overcoming Emotional Eating classes, where my clients also received a lot of benefit from them (in a group setting they are especially powerful). In addition, I shared these methods with some of my friends who were dealing with similar baggage, and they proved useful for them as well.

I tell you this because I want you to know that these assignments didn't just come out of my head to fill up space in a book. Every one of them is a tried-and-true tool, designed to guide you forward on your personal journey.

Two very powerful exercises for healing old hurts are the Releasing Ritual and the Emotional "Enema" Letter. (Maybe we should think of a better name for the second one. Let's call it the Emotional Clearing Letter. I called it the "enema" for two reasons—one, it's good for a laugh when we're about to do some heavy work, and, two, it gets everything out!) There have been some amazing results in our OEE classes when we write these letters. I've seen people let go of many years' worth of suppressed feelings, or get in touch with and release old hurts they didn't even realize they were still carrying. In nearly every case, people report that the emotional baggage they've been carrying seems much lighter afterward.

Here is how it works: First, make a list of people in your life, past or present, who have caused you significant hurts or trauma. We're talking about the kinds of old wounds that still affect you when you think about them. Next, separate the people on this list into two categories. Category one is for people whom you still intend to have some kind of a relationship with (including yourself). We will use the Emotional Clearing Letter for this group.

Category two is for people whom you need to let go of completely, or perhaps who have passed away. We will use the Releasing Ritual for this group.

As you are drawing up your lists, be thorough. Think back through your childhood and forward to the present. It doesn't matter how long ago the hurt occurred; what matters is cleansing the wound so it can heal.

ASSIGNMENT: Emotional Clearing Letter

For each person on the first list, you'll write a separate Emotional Clearing Letter. *Please note that you are **not** to give the letter to the person it is directed toward.* I've had class members write a letter to their ex-spouse, and then, after they have read it to our group and gotten worked up about the situation all over again, they declare, "That $%#&^*@! I'm gonna send this letter, so I can really let it all out!" Please don't. Trust me, it will only open a can of worms and make things worse, because then you'll be hooked back into waiting for their reply and become more emotional, imagining what they'll say and remembering your old hurt over and over—ugh. Just don't. The point of this exercise is to free you from old pain—not reawaken it.

If there are certain categories of people—for example, "everybody who snubbed me because I was overweight"—then go ahead and lump them together into one letter. It can also be very helpful to write a letter to yourself, or to your body. (Later in the chapter I provide an example of a letter I wrote to a part of myself.) If your list is long, don't expect to write all the letters in a day, or even a week.

Emotional Clearing Letters are meant to pull out of you every hidden feeling you have about a person or situation and to shift those feelings toward release and forgiveness. They are meant to help *you* become lighter and freer, *not* to excuse or allow intolerable behavior from others. When I talk about forgiveness, what I mean is for you to be able to release the burden of negative feelings you are carrying toward another person, by and for yourself. *You are not expected to discuss this with them directly or put yourself at risk for any more hurt from them.* This is meant to be a safe, healing process. I repeat, *don't* give this letter to the person you wrote it about! At a later time, if you want to give them an edited version, fine. But not now—this letter is meant for you only, for your healing.

You write the Emotional Clearing Letter by completing a series of sentences that guide you though a variety of emotions—from anger and resentment, to fear, to sadness, and then to your hopes and wishes, and, finally, to feeling love and forgiveness.

Andrea, a woman in one of my classes who'd been through a lot of abuse in her past relationships, was very skeptical about this exercise. She chose her ex-husband as the subject of her first letter. After I explained the assignment, she put her hands on her hips and said sarcastically, "And what—after we write this letter, we're just gonna love the person, huh?"

I replied, "Well, maybe not necessarily *love* him, but at the very least you will let go of some of the junk you've been carrying around about him. So far, he's been living rent free in your head, right? Wouldn't you rather do a little writing work, and evict him?" Now *that* idea she could agree with! And after she completed the exercise, she said that the process helped her let go emotionally and move on with her life.

Using the sentence stems below, write as many statements as you can for each emotion. Don't worry if you have *way* more to write about one particular emotion (like resentments) than another; just be sure to write at least a couple of sentences for each. Stay focused on one person per letter (or, as mentioned above, one group that can be reasonably lumped together). Write it as if you were talking directly to them, saying everything you ever wanted or needed to say to them.

Please don't edit yourself or hold back; just let the feelings and words come out without judgment. No one will see this letter but you and, later, your support person or group. The person in your letter will never see it—they aren't meant to. It's just for you, for your emotional release. If you can allow yourself to experience any feelings you might have as you're writing, all the better, because that's exactly what the process is for.

Dear _____:

I'm still angry about...

I resent the way you...

I wish you had never...

It irritates me that you...

I hate...

(Keep writing on the emotions of anger and resentment until you have nothing left to say on this subject.)

I'm still hurt about...

I feel sad about...

I want to cry whenever I think of...

I wish you had never...

I miss...

Because of these problems, I have lost...

(Keep writing on the emotions of grief and sadness until you have nothing left to say. It's okay to cry, too.)

I'm scared that...

I worry that...

I'm afraid that...

I'm anxious about...

It haunts me that...

(Keep writing out any fearful thoughts and feelings until you don't have anything left to write.)

I regret that I...

I feel really bad that I...

I wish I had never...

I feel guilty about...

I know my part in it was...

(Keep writing until you have listed all your regrets and any personal responsibility you feel about the situation.)

If I had it to do over, I would...

In the future I hope I will...

What I hope for you is...

What I hope for myself is...

I wish...

(Keep writing about your hopes and wishes until you've said all you can.)

I used to love it when...

I did appreciate you for...

I realize that you...

A good thing that came out of it was...

I forgive you for...

I forgive myself for...

There are two final steps that are very important: Please read your letter out loud to someone—but *not* to the person it's written to. Read it to someone neutral, like a sponsor, counselor, or friend. And then burn it.

In my classes, we write the letters as a group, sitting quietly together while each person writes their own; then we read them aloud to each other. This seems scary at first, yet once the first person has read their letter, usually others become willing to read theirs and to release some feelings while receiving the loving support of the group.

People often cry while reading aloud, or even while hearing another's letter. Even though our personal circumstances are different, in many cases the feelings they trigger are the same. By the end of one of these letter-reading classes, our group feels much closer, and each person feels some sense of release—either a little or a lot—from going through the process. Afterward, burning the letter symbolizes closure, really letting it go once and for all, which is explained in detail in the next exercise.

ASSIGNMENT: Releasing Ritual

For this exercise, refer to your second category of people, those whom you need to let go of altogether, people from your past or your present, living or dead. Often we carry emotional ties to past relationships that prevent us from living fully in the present. This letter is designed to cut those ties in a kind but firm manner. Again, the method is to complete the following sentence stems, then read your letter aloud to a trusted friend, and then burn it.

As you burn it, visualize the smoke as your last ties to that person —then watch the smoke evaporate, and affirm that your old baggage is disappearing right along with it. Afterward, you may want to say a prayer, or breathe a few deep, cleansing breaths. As you do this, acknowledge that from this moment forward you are released—free to move on to a more loving, healthy, bountiful life!

Dear _____:

The gifts I received from our time together were...

The gifts I receive from leaving you (or from our parting) are...

The life lessons I learned from our time together were...

What I hope for you is...

What I hope for myself is...

I release you, _____. I completely cut the physical, emotional, mental, and spiritual cords between us. I release you and I release myself, to live a free, happy, and healthy life from now on!

◎   ◎   ◎

Previously I said I'd give you an example of one of my own letters. Many of us have found it surprisingly useful to write one or both of these letters to parts of ourselves—like your inner food addict, or the "gobble gremlin," as I like to call it. Here is a letter I wrote to mine:

Dear Part of Me That Always Wants to Overeat,

The gifts I received from our time together were: You gave me comfort when I was in pain; you gave me a kind of nurturing when I was lonely or frustrated or hurting. You gave me something to look forward to when I didn't know how to fill my time, or at the end of a hard day. You helped me get to sleep when I couldn't. You kept me overweight, which kept away dangerous men. You kept me in hiding a lot of the time because I didn't want to face rejection, then you comforted me with more food when I was lonely and isolated. You helped me to numb out when my feelings were too painful to deal with. You've been a buffer zone between me and life since I was a little girl.

The gifts I've received from leaving you are: Loss of over one hundred pounds, and the return of my overall good health. Being a lot more willing to step up to the plate, face risks and challenges, and thereby accomplish many of my dreams and goals. Feeling better about myself, more energetic, more positive. Enjoying a lot more positive attention from just about everybody, instead of sneers and contempt due to my body size. More opportunities in life, work, and love, including the "opportunity" to face and deal with the issues that were hidden underneath the food, and to clear and release them once and for all, so I can live a healthier life from now on.

The life lessons I learned from my time with you have been: Realizing I have paid a heavy price for avoiding my feelings by using food. Every time I gave in to your desire to overeat, I got fatter, more depressed, and more stuck. And while that was going on, many years of my life slipped away. The lesson is to make loving choices for my health today, right now, so I can feel good about me inside and out.

What I hope for you is: I hope that the real you, my hungry and hurting inner child, will receive the steadfast love and nurturing she needs, not from excess food or from men—but from me, from my making better choices about how I nurture her. As long as I give her real love, and listen to and care for her needs, she won't need to overeat anymore.

What I hope for myself is: I hope to take good care of my body, heart, and spirit, so that I can finally let go of using food as an option for dealing with my feelings. I hope to be free to live my dreams, and to encourage others to do the same—starting right now!

Inner Child Work

Using the letter-writing method to heal and release previous traumas is just one of many tools available for clearing away old baggage. Inner child work and family of origin work can also be very helpful. If you're unfamiliar with these concepts, here's the basic idea: Each of us has a wounded inner child who never healed from early trauma we experienced. It's as if, even though our bodies grew up and became adults, there is still a part of us that is emotionally stuck at age three or five or eight—depending on how old we were when certain traumas or tragedies happened to us. The child inside us is still hurting and needs our help in order to heal and move on.

In our families, we may have been neglected or abused in a variety of ways. This doesn't mean that our parents were bad people; they may have been very good people who were just doing the best they could with what they had to give. According to John Bradshaw, one of the leading authorities in this field, nearly everyone has experienced at least some verbal or emotional wounding during their early years, whether from their parents or from other adult caretakers, like teachers, babysitters, coaches, or religious figures.

Our inner child, trying to make sense of these hurts but lacking the power of adult reasoning, made incorrect decisions about life, ourselves, and other people. These decisions hardened into beliefs over the years, contaminating and sabotaging our lives as adults. For example, a child who experienced a lot of abuse from a parent might decide "It's not safe to love anybody," or "You can't trust love," or, worse, "Love is supposed to hurt."

Unless we really go deep within to reprogram and heal our inner child, beliefs like these might lead us into relationships with abusive partners, or they might cause us to avoid getting close to anyone for fear of being hurt again. This keeps us stuck, living out our old patterns, and the hurt or loneliness we feel as a result may trigger us into overeating.

How do you know if you have a traumatized inner child who is sabotaging your life? Here are some clues:

- You have a history of abuse or neglect (physical, verbal, emotional, or sexual) as a child or teenager.
- You have a history of difficulty in personal relationships, whether with family, friends, coworkers, or loved ones.
- You have a tendency to overreact in close relationships whenever any problems or miscommunications arise.
- You have a fear of abandonment, which is an excessive fear of losing someone you love, a fear of their leaving you.
- You have a fear of engulfment, which is a fear of being trapped or smothered, an excessive fear of closeness.
- You feel excessively deep pain and grief—as though you've been "kicked in the gut"—whenever there's a problem in a relationship.
- You feel an overwhelming, gut-wrenching fear and anxiety—almost terror—over relationship problems.
- You do just about anything to avoid this deep pain or terror.

If we have these issues, how do we heal them? The answer, like many I've offered, involves some good news and some "other" news. Some of this healing may involve going back in time, through visualization or hypnosis, to contact the part of yourself that experienced the original trauma, to reparent yourself through the situation, and to change the negative beliefs that originated back then into positive ones. Other methods include visualization, writing about the traumatic incident with your nondominant hand (meaning if you're right-handed, use your left hand, and vice versa), and memory anchoring.

To those of you who may be thinking that this whole "inner child" thing is a bunch of new-age foolishness, I have this to say: Just try it. Try using some of the methods listed here, and a bevy of deep feelings may come out, feelings that you didn't even know were still inside of you.

But I won't lie to you. Doing this work isn't easy. You may feel emotionally drained or vulnerable while you're doing it, and sometimes for hours afterward.

So right about here you may be wondering, "If it's that uncomfortable to do this, then what's the payoff in dredging up all that old stuff?" Actually, there's a lot of benefit to it. You'll begin to feel freer, lighter, more energetic, less fatigued, less depressed, less irritable, and more confident. Once this healing work is done, you'll stop sabotaging yourself, and your positive changes will stand a much better chance of lasting for the rest of your life!

And here's another positive: Not all of the time you spend nurturing your inner child has to involve emotional work. What is any child's favorite thing to do? Play! So instead of just doing inner child "work," you can balance it out with an equal measure of inner child "play." You get to enjoy some agenda-free playtime, whether that means going to the beach, playing with arts and crafts, going to the zoo, taking a fun hike, or watching a Disney movie. It really isn't that important what you do, as long as it's something your "inner kid" loves to do. Be sure to carve out a couple of hours for play on a regular basis.

Addressing the full range of inner child work, and the corresponding methods of healing and reparenting, is beyond the scope of this book, but if any of the symptoms on the above list ring true for you, then I highly encourage you to look into it further. Some excellent sources for inner child work are listed in the Resources section located at the back of the book.

chapter
nine

Overcoming
Obstacles
along the Way
Stuck Points, Sabotage,
and Other Addictions

Still overeating?
What's eating you?

Sometimes it can be hard to follow any kind of program that calls for change, such as the one outlined in this book. If you find that's the case for you, never fear. This chapter is devoted to troubleshooting some of the issues that may cause you to experience difficulties.

If you've been looking at your program as a strict boot-camp kind of discipline that you *must* follow perfectly, but you've had some slips, chances are you're feeling disappointed or frustrated with yourself. I encourage you to take a different view: to look at your program as a refuge, a way to buffer the scrapes and scratches you encounter in daily life. In the past, we used food as a way to "take the edge off" certain feelings or situations; then we paid the price with added pounds, guilt, and remorse.

Now, with practice, you will find that your new set of tools—such as sharing your feelings with a friend, journaling, praying, or even a bubble bath—will give you an even better, more substantial relief than food ever could. And with no calories or guilt!

In this chapter we will revisit your body, your heart, and your mind, as well as your social life and relationships, and we will introduce some ideas for dealing with common problems people have when they're changing how they relate to food. No system works perfectly all the time, because there will always be exceptions to the rules. Even when you're in the groove and moving along smoothly, life challenges can arise and knock you off balance. Keep in mind that your program is only a guideline to steer by and a way to realign yourself when you get off track.

Also keep in mind that just as no program is perfect, none of us are perfect, either. We do the best we can on any given day, and some days are better than others, right? When learning to live with your new, improved eating and health habits, the results you get may be hampered by a variety of issues, such as whether or not you have health concerns, take certain medications, have mental health-issues like depression or anxiety—and whether or not your relationships, past and present, may be sabotaging your progress.

If you're experiencing difficulties in following your new eating and exercise plan, here are some general pointers:

o **Don't beat yourself up.** Remember, being mean to yourself has never helped you to achieve any long-lasting goals, has it? So please don't go there. Instead, just tell yourself, "So I got off track. Now I'm going to love myself enough to do what it takes to get back on track."

o **Take small, consistent steps to refocus yourself on your program.** Often our guilty reaction to getting off track is to swing all the way in the other direction—for example, "I over-ate yesterday, so I'll starve myself today." This method rarely works, and besides, you didn't sin, so you don't need to punish yourself. Just get back on track as soon as you recognize the problem. Which brings me to the next point.

o **Stay out of denial by using a food log, scale, and journal.** It's so easy to take a bite of this and a bite of that without even realizing it. Or to say, "I'll exercise tomorrow." Pretty soon a week has passed, you're out of the groove, and where did those five pounds come from? If you keep track of what you're eating, what you weigh, and what's happening in your life day-by-day, within a week you'll see clearly what is really going on. Otherwise, our minds tend to cloud things over, to pretend we're doing things differently than we really are. Use concrete tools to see what's really happening; then you can decide how to deal with it.

o **Take an inventory of your problem areas.** Once you get a clearer picture of what's really going on with you and your food, look over the times and situations when you tend to get off track with your eating. Is it usually evening snacking? Or when you experience a particular feeling? Are certain kinds of foods calling your name? Getting clear about your high-risk areas will help you develop a prevention plan for next time.

o **Most important, don't give up!** So many times in the past I'd use my "slips" as a way to justify *really* going off my food plan.

I'd tell myself, "Well, I already blew it today, so I might as well just go for it. I'll start again tomorrow." I don't know about you, but for me it has never been easy to stop a food binge once I get started. It's better to stop with the first little slip, before it picks up speed. Don't give up!

Now it's time to get specific. Let's look at possible problem areas one by one.

Physical Stuck Points
◎

There are a variety of reasons why your body may not be responding as well as you'd like to your nutrition and exercise plan. Among these are physical problems that may restrict your ability to exercise, certain medications, and dietary restrictions caused by health concerns. Although this is by no means a comprehensive list, some of the medications that can inhibit weight loss are insulin, hormone therapies, and certain antidepressants. Let's look at some examples...

◎ Eva's Story

Eva, a thirty-five-year-old diabetic mother of three, was in a preoperative screening program for weight loss surgery when she began attending my classes. Although I emphasize consuming primarily proteins, vegetables, amino acids, and multivitamin supplements, I am always careful to tell my clients to check with their physician prior to implementing any of these changes.

After consulting her doctor, Eva came back to class disappointed. "My doctor said that because of my kidney and liver problems, I'm not supposed to eat all that protein or take the amino acids," she said. But because she had diabetes, the fact that the plan suggested a low carbohydrate intake and avoidance of sugar was a real plus. We worked together to develop a variety of meal plans

(cont'd.)

that suited her lifestyle. We emphasized soups, stews, salads, lots of fresh veggies, and a moderate amount of protein.

Eva also had some serious challenges when it came to movement and exercise. She weighed over three hundred pounds, and her hips, knees, and ankles hurt whenever she'd try to walk for any distance. But she didn't give up, and eventually she discovered water exercise. Soon she was going to the beach three times a week with her family and moving around in the buoyant salt water, where she could stretch her body and improve her circulation without putting any stress on her joints.

Of course, not everyone lives near a beach, but water exercise is a great alternative for anyone whose limitations prevent them from engaging in weight-bearing activities such as walking or hiking. Most areas have either a nearby gym or a YMCA with a swimming pool that offers water aerobics classes; at the very least, try the open-swim time if the classes aren't to your liking. The point is, don't let your limitations stop you; get creative, like Eva did, and find a way to move that works for you.

Other physical limitations may include debilitating injuries, certain medications that inhibit weight loss, hormonal changes that cause food cravings, or a combination of all of the above.

◎ Mindy's Story

Mindy, a forty-five-year-old landscape designer, had lived most of her life at a normal weight, until she was in an accident that damaged her spine. Since then she'd had to be very careful to prevent any further injury, and as a result she was no longer able to hike, scuba dive, or do any of the outdoor activities she enjoyed.

These restrictions bore some serious consequences. Within a year she'd gained fifty pounds, and she became very depressed due to her weight and her physical limitations. Around the same time, she also began to experience premenopausal symptoms such as mood swings, night sweats, and frequent evening cravings for sweets and starches. Her depression became serious enough that she consulted her doctor, who put her on antidepressant medication and recommended hormone-replacement therapy.

These medications did help Mindy's depression, and gradually, as her overall mood improved, she was able to investigate alternative forms of exercise. She found that slow walks on a flat track didn't hurt her back; eventually she bought a treadmill, which she uses at least three times per week. She studied alternative hormone-replacement therapies and began using amino acids and other herbal supplements, which helped to lessen her symptoms. As a result of these changes, Mindy stopped the evening snacking, felt better from exercising several times per week, dropped some weight, and returned to a happier, healthier state of mind.

More and more research is finding that many of the traits that used to be taken for granted as simply part of one's personality or the result of moods in fact have a basis in body chemistry. This is good news for overeaters, for as long as we are willing to adjust our intake of food and nutritional supplements, and to find creative ways to keep striving for a better quality of life, we *can* overcome these physical obstacles to maintaining a healthy body weight.

Mental and Emotional Stuck Points

Certain thoughts and feelings can sabotage us, draining our motivation to follow through with our program. Maybe you harbor thoughts like, "What's the use, anyway? I'll never get this right, so I might as well enjoy myself and eat _____." Or maybe you live with feelings of depression or even hopelessness. In my journal entries I call these the "demons" that try to talk me out of making healthy choices, and I do my best to resist them.

There is also a rebellious, childish part of me that I jokingly call my "inner brat." She is about three years old and doesn't care at all about things like numbers on a bathroom scale or long-term success. She only knows what she wants *right now*. And she is likely to have a power tantrum to get it. You know those kids in the check-out line at the market, yelling their heads off because they want some goodie they see? That's my inner brat. If I let her win, if I give in to her because I'm tired or frustrated or it just seems like the path of least resistance, then the next time she knows she can get away with it and she yells even louder.

And there are also plain old bad habits—things we've done a certain way for so many years that now we do them on autopilot, like eating as a knee-jerk reaction to stress or boredom, or being triggered to overeat merely by seeing or talking about food. How do we change a habit? The answer is simple, but not easy. We change a habit gradually, every time we make a different choice, and by recognizing that each of these positive choices for our health, no matter how seemingly small, helps us to create a *new* habit—one we want, instead of one we don't want.

Do you have an inner brat, or some entrenched bad habits? Or an infestation of the gloom-and-doom demons who tell you that you'll never make it, so why try? If so, it's important to find a way to shut them up. Luckily, there are some tried-and-true methods we can use.

One such method again involves dealing with your body chemistry. If you drink plenty of water and eat small meals of protein and veggies three to five times daily, your fatigue and depression may improve greatly. If this isn't enough, amino acid supplementation has proved helpful for many in balancing brain chemistry. You'd be surprised at how many of our thoughts and feelings are influenced by an imbalance of neurotransmitters in the brain. A lack of serotonin, for instance, can cause worry, anxiety, obsessive negative thoughts, and depression. A lack of norepinephrine can cause us to feel overly sensitive, flat, joyless, or like there's no love in our lives—so we'd better eat some chocolate! One solution may be to take supplements of amino acids or other herbs that raise bodily levels of these neurotransmitters, if these are appropriate for you and meet with your doctor's approval. To increase serotonin levels, you can take 5-HTP or L-tryptophan, or the herb St. John's wort. To increase norepinephrine, take DLPA, also known as DL-phenylalanine. Another amino acid, L-glutamine, is useful for balancing blood sugar and can help reduce many types of food cravings. Specific recommended dosages are listed in Appendix A, located at the back of the book. I can almost guarantee you that one of these will help raise your mood—and they're calorie free!

You may also wish to consider using positive affirmations in a very targeted way. You may have heard that affirmations are just a bunch of airy-fairy, New-Age foolishness, but it ain't true. Yes, they are a form of brainwashing, but sometimes our brain *needs* a good washing! How many times have we gotten upset or fearful over all the "what-ifs" churning through our mind? Maybe we even tell people what we are worrying about, and the more we say it, the more we believe it. This is called "awfulizing"—taking a grain of truth and magnifying it into a big imaginary problem. Isn't this a form of using our thoughts and words to affect how we feel—but negatively so? And haven't we all done this?

My point is that using affirmations isn't something new. It's just taking conscious control of a process that has already been going on below the surface of the mind. Using affirmations turns our mind in the direction we want it to go, instead of letting it control us like a runaway horse.

Whatever negative messages your brain is sending you, you can figure out some positive alternatives to them. Write, say, or listen to them *often,* preferably daily. For example, perhaps your "demons" say stuff like "You'll never look great no matter what you weigh," or "You're too old/ugly/screwed up, so what difference does it make if you eat a lot?" Whenever you catch messages such as these flitting through your mind, replace them with new messages like "I deserve to be the best I can be," or "I am a precious, beautiful child of God," or "Real self-love means taking good care of my body." Or come up with your own positive messages, as we discussed in Chapter 5.

Yes, I know it sounds corny. Yes, I know you may feel uncomfortable or even silly saying these things. So what? If you are letting your negative self-talk get the better of you and it is sabotaging your program, then it's in your best interest to be open-minded about possible solutions, especially if what you've been doing so far hasn't been working very well.

An even better method of using affirmations is to make an audio recording of your favorites and listen to them whenever you can. I used to have a forty-five-minute commute to work every day, and during the drive I would make myself crazy with a bunch of negative "what-ifs" about my job, my partner, you name it. I'd get myself all worked up, and then I'd arrive at work in a funk. Once I became aware of this pattern, I decided to do something about it. Using the guidelines I am about to give you, I made some personalized cassette tapes of positive affirmations, set to soothing background music. Guess what? After listening to those tapes in my car for just a couple of months, the negative voices retreated, I felt better, and my thoughts turned in a more positive direction. In other words—it worked!

How to Customize Positive Affirmations

First, listen to the negative voices in your head and write down what they're saying. No, I don't think you're crazy or hearing voices. But most people have an internal monologue that goes on below the surface all the time. You could be driving down the road on your way to work and it might be saying something like this:

"When I get to work, I've got to do _____, and I'd better hurry up and finish before the boss gives me a hard time. God knows **I've had enough hard times** with my boyfriend and my kids over the past few days. Seems like **there's always one more problem**—I don't need any more of that right now. Why do they always blame me? Feels like **no matter how hard I try, I'm never good enough.** You'd think people could look at their own side of the street, but no. **I always get the blame,** and then **everybody puts me down.** I hate it. Wonder what there is to eat in the fridge at work. Maybe I should get some pastry now, just in case...."

Sound familiar? The words in boldface are the kinds of negative statements I'm talking about. Usually we don't even realize we're saying these things to ourselves, yet unconsciously we are allowing a negative set of beliefs to become ingrained—beliefs that can sabotage our every effort to feel good. Yet for every negative there's a positive, and once you uncover your own "negative affirmations" you have a golden opportunity to retrain, rewire, and reorganize your brain in a very specific way.

Using the statements above, let's try some examples:

Positive Affirmations that Counter Negative Self-Talk

Negative self-talk	Positive affirmations
I've had enough hard times.	My life is flowing along happily, smoothly, and easily.
There's always one more problem.	I meet new challenges successfully and with ease.
No matter how hard I try, I'm never good enough.	I'm valuable and lovable just as I am right now. I'm good enough just as I am.
I always get the blame.	I am treated with respect and kindness.
Everybody puts me down.	Lots of people love and appreciate me.

This is just one possible scenario. I encourage you to play detective with your own internal monologue, figure out what your inner voices are saying, and come up with some simple, present-tense affirmations to counter them. Try recording your affirmations on a tape or CD. In this way, you can listen to them in the car or whenever you have some private time. They've worked for me and for many others!

Social and Interpersonal Stuck Points

◎

When my personal relationships are going smoothly, it's fairly easy for me to stick to my food plan. But when I'm having trouble with loved ones, friends, family, or even coworkers, it becomes more of a challenge. It's so easy to get thrown off balance when someone treats us poorly. Many overeaters report being especially sensitive in this area, and I'm no exception. I wish I had a thicker skin when it comes to my relationships—but I don't.

Lacking that, I try to do the next best thing: to surf the emotional waves instead of getting pounded by them. I use my recovery tools to help me stay on an even keel, to remind me not to take everything so personally, to attempt to let things flow "like water off a duck's back." It's not always easy, but it is worth it. Sometimes the leftover boogeymen from all those years of being fat get in my way. I used to think I needed to stay in relationships even when I was being treated poorly, because some part of me remained stuck in believing no one would want me. It's crazy-making—and when I hurt enough to recognize it, I do something about it.

When we find ourselves in pain that's triggered by a relationship, it's important to figure out what's causing it. Am I hurting because I've been treated disrespectfully? Then I need to communicate this to the other person, and perhaps set some boundaries around what kind of treatment I will and will not accept. Many times this will be enough to work out the problem, but sometimes we have to have this discussion more than once. We may need to negotiate our boundaries, especially around issues like time and money.

One of my best friends, Lisa, lives by a very different inner clock than I do. She probably considers me to be a little on the frantic side, and I secretly consider her to be in slow motion. If we didn't love and respect each other so much, if we didn't have so many other good things in common, we might not even be friends. But we are, so we have learned to work around the timing. We talked about it, and we both moved a little toward the middle. I eased up on being driven by the clock, and she became a little more aware of it. As a result, our friendship has survived and flourished for many years. Issues such as these become a little trickier in a love relationship, but they can still be worked through. Doing so may just take a little more compassion and detachment.

Another area where we may need to set boundaries is with people who tempt us to overeat. When I was a drug abuse counselor, part of my job was to warn my newly clean and sober clients to be very careful around their old drug addict friends, because those were the very people most likely to tempt them back into their old habits with alcohol and drugs.

Avoiding these people seems like common sense when it comes to staying off drugs—yet how many times have supposedly well-meaning friends and loved ones pushed a piece of pie into your face, saying, "Go ahead, have some! Just a little won't hurt you!" And the tricky thing is that since food is so much more socially acceptable than drugs, it's easy to let down our guard and allow them to talk us into it. Especially after you've lost weight and look "normal," it's important to remember where you came from so you'll stay on track. Don't let those normal eaters tempt you into thinking you are just like them. Even after losing the weight, if you aren't careful you may still be susceptible to old habits that can lead to weight gain.

A Spy in the House of Thin

At one year post-op, I'd lost a hundred pounds. On the inside, I was much the same person I'd always been. Of course, as I replaced my old habits with healthier ones, I felt better about myself—but my personality was the same, my history and experiences were the same, my essence, the core of who I was, remained unchanged.

But on the outside, whew! Everything was different. Because my body looked better, all of a sudden I was receiving tons of positive attention. People who had known me before now treated me with so much complimentary approval it was almost embarrassing.

Men who had never given me the time of day were suddenly asking me out, opening doors for me, making small talk. Women were asking me to lunch. People in general smiled and were nice to me, instead of avoiding eye contact. After many years of my being sneered at and jeered at because of my weight, you'd think all this would make me happy, right?

Well, sometimes it did. I mean, who could resist being treated with kindness instead of rejection? Of course it felt better! But sometimes, especially when it came from people who had ignored me when I was big, it left me feeling kind of sick inside.

The other day I ran into a man who was my neighbor a few years ago. He'd always been distantly friendly toward me, never mean—but he really had the hots for my roommate, a pretty woman with long blond hair who rebuffed him repeatedly. He'd go on and on to me about how beautiful she was, and he'd ask if I could help him get a date with her. I remember wondering if he had the least bit of awareness, even a shred of sensitivity, about how this made me feel, like I was some sexless lump who shouldn't even *dream* of being wanted by a man.

When I saw him recently, he gave me a big hug and wanted to know all about how I was doing. "And by the way, are you seeing anybody?" he said, as his eyes moved over my new figure. I muttered something noncommittal, but he pushed his card into my hand anyway. "Call me sometime—you never know," he said, smiling and standing a little too close.

I took the card, said goodbye, and made my escape. I dropped the card on the ground as I got into my car and made a point to run over it as I drove away. "Yeah, you never know," I said aloud with irritation. "You never know when you're being an insensitive jerk, I guess."

Whatever.

It just hurts sometimes.

Looking like everybody else on the outside yet still feeling like a fat person on the inside has been a peculiar experience. I feel like a spy in the thin world, like I'm passing for normal—but I've put the situation to good use. When someone tells a fat joke or makes a judgmental remark about an overweight person, I take the opportunity to educate them about fat prejudice. They're surprised at first, but after they've heard a brief version of my story, they usually seem a little more open-minded and willing to look at their own attitudes. I hope they get it.

On another memorable occasion, I attempted to fight off a nation-wide craze that finally found its way to Maui—Krispy Kreme Donuts. I felt like the only bird flying north when everybody else was flying south—but I managed.

Why Krispy Kreme Is the Devil

An island is a small place, like a country village in many ways. Life can be pretty slow, so when anything new happens, however small, it's a big deal to the locals. I remember my surprise at the hoopla generated by the opening of our K-Mart outlet a few years ago. I mean, come on, it's only a store, right? But it was a very big deal on Maui!

Still, nothing could have prepared me for the collective near-frenzy that erupted over the arrival of the island's first Krispy Kreme donut shop. Its coming was heralded with all the fanfare that would accompany a visiting dignitary. The radio stations, newspapers, and television stations got caught up in the general furor over these hot-off-the-conveyer-belt delicacies. Radio announcers offered free dozens to faithful listeners, and one local newspaper had a big taste test—the prize being, of course, more Krispy Kreme donuts.

The night before their grand opening, people actually camped out in front of the store like it was a Rolling Stones concert. On opening day, the police had to be called in to direct the volumes of traffic headed into the store. This went on for the next several days. Krispy Kreme was on everyone's lips, literally and otherwise. In the bank, in the grocery store, at work—it seemed like no matter where I went, someone was saying, "Have you tried the new Krispy Kremes yet?" and someone else was replying, "Oh my God, aren't they great?"

I tried my best to avoid these conversations, especially when they degraded into passionate, graphic descriptions of the creme-filled this or the chocolate-covered that, lustful odes to the donuts' glazed and powdered exteriors. I really didn't want to hear it. I've listened to many of my addict clients describe their favorite drug in loving detail—how it looked, what it tasted like, how good it made them feel. Often they could recall the smell, taste, and feel of the drug long after their last run. And I can't help but see the similarities between the drug addict and the Krispy Kreme convert. Ever since that evil place opened, all I've been hearing is how people will drive miles out of their way to get their donut "fix," how they will eat several at one sitting, how they feel a little sick afterward but can't wait to do it again. Ugh.

Night before last, I went to a new writer's meeting for the first time. During the break, a big blond lady wearing gold earrings and a tight pink sweater came up to me with a plate of donuts. She held it only a few inches from my face. "These are from Krispy Kreme," she said. "They're really great—try some," as she pushed the plate invitingly under my nose.

The donuts' wet, sweet, yeasty fragrance curled up into my face. A welcoming light seemed to sparkle from their crystalline, sugary surface. I looked longingly at them, and they seemed to look seductively back at me.

"No thanks," I managed to reply. "I don't eat sugar or wheat anymore." I didn't bother to explain further.

A slightly confused frown creased her cheerful face. "Oh—well, you can still have just one, right? One can't hurt you." She continued to hold the plate under my nose.

"Well, I've lost over a hundred pounds and kept it off for some time now by *not* eating that stuff—so I really don't want any, thanks."

"Hey, that's really great—over a hundred pounds? You don't look like you've ever been fat—you sure you don't want to try just a little?"

She still hadn't moved the plate, so this time my tone was a bit sharper. "No, thanks, " I said. "Could you *take* those things away from me, please?" She finally lowered the plate, looking a tad offended, and walked off, presumably to find easier prey.

Oh well. It wasn't the first time. Last week, in my Overcoming Emotional Eating class, I managed to upset a group member who was going on about how wonderful the Krispy Kremes were. I interrupted her with, "Can we please not go there, for my sake and for the rest of the class?" She, too, looked offended, but she shut up. Really, what worse place to sing donut love songs than in a class like that?

I guess I am not exactly winning friends lately by setting these boundaries, but I feel I have to protect myself. For people like me—compulsive overeaters who would surely set off a binge by eating "just one" of those donuts—they're like the devil, whispering promises of a quick feel-good fix, then stealing your health and peace of mind once you're hooked. I don't want to see them, I don't want to smell them, and I definitely don't want to hear about how great they supposedly are. Having spent most of my life as a slave to sugar cravings, I am, in fact, a little afraid of them—my relatively new size-six figure notwithstanding.

◎   ◎   ◎

Yet what about those times when it's not an issue of what the rest of the world is doing, or how "they" are treating me? What if the source of the problem is how needy or sensitive *I'm* feeling? As we discussed in Chapter 8, sometimes old baggage or unhealed wounds from past relationships can influence how we interpret events in our present-day lives. If we are seeing things negatively, it may trigger us to overeat.

◎ Fred's Story

Fred is a handsome thirty-four-year-old chef with a passion for horses, a talent for guitar, and a strong desire to find his soul mate and settle down. After losing eighty-five pounds from WLS a few years ago, he feels ready, willing, and able to find a partner. Yet despite his good looks, great career, and kind heart, he is almost always single. He has a very suspicious side to his personality, which may be a result of his having been through a lot of rough times growing up. As a kid, he was abused and abandoned over and over by his alcoholic mother, and he learned to protect himself with a tough exterior, and with overeating to dull the pain.

Now, unfortunately, he sees shadows from his past in every corner, and he sees a "witch" in every woman he meets. Maybe some of the women he's been with did treat him poorly, but some of them have been really great ladies—only Fred can't see that. He's too busy seeing their every action as a repeat of his mother's abandonment from his childhood. They try to get close to him, but they can't get through his hard, protective shell. Eventually they give up and leave, and he says, "See? I was right. Just another bimbo!"

Can you see how, at least to some degree, it's Fred's own attitude and his own fears causing these problems?

Dealing with deep-seated issues like these may require a multidimensional solution. Affirmations can be very useful, along with awareness of your "ghosts" and how they may be affecting your life today. If this isn't enough, and it may not be, then consider getting individual or family therapy and working out your issues on a deeper level with some expert guidance.

Environmental Stuck Points

◎

I feel blessed to live in what is an ideal physical environment for me. Not only do I live on Maui, Hawaii, but I have the luxury of a temptation-free environment most of the time. My home is peaceful, and—wonder of wonders—there's no junk food in it! There are also no sugar or wheat products or any of the other binge foods that I prefer to avoid. None of it is in my home. I am so grateful for that.

But it wasn't always this way, believe me. For most of my life, keeping all my "comfort foods" around was how I felt safe and secure. If I had a craving for, say, a chocolate-chip cookie, I'd buy a whole bag of them. After I'd eaten my fill for the moment, they were still there, so of course I'd have to eat the rest! I couldn't just throw them away, could I? Multiply this by lots of cravings over many years, and there you have one of my biggest triggers: a houseful of junk food that I couldn't throw away or say no to. Many of my diets were sabotaged simply by having junk food in the house.

Finally, I realized that living this way wasn't working for me. After my weight loss surgery, I asked the people around me to please support me in making a change to a trigger-free, junk-free environment. Initially I was pretty hard-core about not wanting anything questionable in the house, but after about sixteen months I felt strong enough to compromise. Although "the other people's food" (that's how I think of it) was no longer totally absent, my roommates did agree to keep it out of sight in a separate cabinet or container somewhere so I didn't ever have to see it. That proved to be enough—as long as I didn't go snooping in drawers and cabinets where the trigger food was hiding!

If part of your problem with overeating involves being triggered by seeing certain foods, smelling them, or just knowing they're there— get rid of them. If you can't totally get rid of them because they belong to someone else, hopefully you can convince your loved ones to at least store them out of sight.

Spiritual Stuck Points
◎

A lack of purpose, a sense of emptiness, feeling scattered, feeling lost— all these can come from neglecting our spiritual practices or never using them regularly to begin with. Maybe we went through bad experiences early on with "the God thing" and don't want anything to do with it now. Yet haven't we often made food our "higher power" by using it to relieve stress or problems we didn't know how to solve?

There's an old saying: "When you feel far away from God, guess who moved?" It's not that you're doing anything wrong; it's just that you haven't made this aspect of your life a priority. Making time for spiritual development may sound like a good idea, but who has the time? We may agree that it's important—yet never do it. We just carry on with the necessary tasks of the day, the week, the year.... The only problem is, the empty feeling keeps returning.

I encourage you to take the time—to *make* the time—to utilize some of the methods outlined in Chapter 7 for developing a spiritual practice, even if only for ten minutes at a time, three or four days a week. You may be surprised by how much even this little bit of spiritual focus can do to increase your serenity and sense of purpose.

◎   ◎   ◎

Wherever you find yourself getting stuck—whether in habits of body, mind, or spirit—just know that it is a normal part of the process of change. Don't beat yourself up or give up too soon. There are solutions. It takes time to learn new skills and habits. Nobody does it perfectly!

Keep doing the best you can to find creative ways to get over, under, and around your roadblocks, and you'll get there. If you do get stuck in the muck, never fear. Here's how I pulled myself out of it and launched myself back into my recovery.

Dwelling on the Threshold

By seven months after weight loss surgery I had already lost seventy-five pounds. I was involved in a support group, and I ate no junk food, no starch, and no sugar. I took my vitamins and proteins, and I exercised three times a week. I'd gone back to meditating several times a week and praying every day. But my weight loss had slowed way down, whereas before it had been easy. And the appetite I'd been so relieved to get rid of was starting to reappear, to my great dismay.

If there was any value in my struggle—if there were any lessons to be learned from the "one step forward, two steps back" kind of progress I seemed to be making—well, I sure wanted to learn them and get on with it! Take a look at any media output, from TV to magazines, from movies to some self-help books, and you'll find that nobody tells you about the struggle part. If it's on TV, the drama is resolved in under an hour. If it's one of those late-night infomercials trying to get you to buy something, they always show you the "before" and "after" pictures, but they never show the "during" pictures, the messy daily battle that really goes on inside a person who's trying to change.

The "in-between" part is not exciting or particularly newsworthy. The photos that show fat to thin, flabby to buff, bald to a youthful head of hair—those are dramatic enough to get the desperate and the hopeful on the phone with their credit cards. But if the pill, or the machine, or the promises are so great, why are advertisers spending big bucks to seduce you through the TV? Why do their dramatic stories always come with fine print that says "results not typical"?

In some cases I think it's because their products are a bunch of junk, but in some cases maybe the product isn't the problem. Maybe the "problem" (which isn't necessarily a problem) lies with us humans. Change tends to sound a lot easier than it actually is. Change requires more of us than staying in our familiar rut does.

Speaking for myself, my struggles to avoid overeating, to deal with problems as they arise, to face my fears of risk and rejection—well, they haven't been easy. Every day is full of little choices. Each choice I make to evolve—to exercise, to meditate, to step out of my comfort zone and try new things—breathes life into the person I am becoming. And every choice I make to fall back into procrastination, hiding, and nibbling reinforces the old habit monster that I want to starve to death.

If you've spent thirty years being fat, like I did, you know the pain of rejection all too well. We've all heard stories of the abused dog or cat who lived its life in a tiny cage, then was finally set free—*only to confine itself to living in a similarly small part of the house, because that limited space was all it knew.* We've heard the stories and we understand the parable. We get it that change is difficult. So why don't we cut ourselves a little more slack, be a little kinder to ourselves as we go through this process?

The return of the gastric bypass patient's appetite at approximately six months to one year post-op is such a common pattern that it's become a standard part of the WLS literature. All the surgery veterans told me it would happen—but I didn't really believe them. They told me that their struggles with appetite got worse and worse, until some of them gave in to their appetites and gained much of their weight back.

Others, like me, stalled out well above their ideal weight and now battled cravings every day. They maintained a good weight loss overall—many had lost over a hundred pounds—but they weren't free. The bag of cookies in the kitchen was still calling their name. And although my overweight friends and I used to laugh about stuff like that, I wasn't laughing anymore. I'd come too far. There was no way I was going to go through what remained of my life overweight, still struggling with food cravings the way an addict struggles to stay clean. That was no kind of freedom, no kind of life. I wanted to be free.

I *want* to be free.

ASSIGNMENT: Is It Food Addiction?

Many people are uncomfortable using the word "addiction" when it comes to their eating behavior. And, in fact, it may not apply to you. Here are some medically recognized guidelines to help you determine whether or not your issues with food have crossed the line into addictive behavior. A caution: If you answer yes to three or more of these questions, an indication of addiction, *please* don't beat yourself up. Knowledge about yourself is always helpful, provided you use it in a gentle and loving manner.

1. Do cravings for food occupy your thoughts for a significant portion of each day?

2. Do you often plan and look forward to what yummy food you will have at the end of the day?

3. Has your overeating caused problems with your health, your goals, your self-esteem, or your relationships, and yet you continue to overeat anyway?

4. Have you repeatedly promised yourself that you would cut back or stop overeating, but find it hard to stick to your promises?

5. Do you find that when you eat certain foods (like sweets, fried foods, or starches), that once you have a little bit it's hard to stop?

6. Do you find that when you try to cut those "trigger" foods out of your diet, you get cranky and crave them until you give in and go back to eating them?

7. Do you sometimes hide your overeating from others so you can eat more without being observed? For instance, maybe you stay up late to indulge, or eat in the car, or eat while "cleaning up" after dinner or a party.

8. Do you sometimes eat past the point of fullness (i.e., keep eating even though your tummy is stuffed)?

9. Have you frequently waged an internal battle by thinking, "I've really got to stop doing this to myself"—yet you keep overeating anyway?

10. Does living life with three medium-sized, low-starch, no-sugar meals daily seem really boring or unpleasant?

Again, if you answered yes to three or more of the above questions, don't feel bad. I answered yes to all of them! And yet I have still managed to find a way to live a rich, satisfying life without excess food—and so can you.

Even if you've answered yes to three or more and are now considering the idea that part of your problem has been food addiction, never fear. Addiction has both physical and psychological components that can be successfully addressed using the methods provided throughout this book. Another way to lessen the stigma of the word "addiction" is to remember that even if we are food addicts, we aren't bad people; we were simply using the best coping skill available to us at the time. And now that we know better, hopefully we can do better.

Those of us who have lived with a large enough body size that we qualified for this life-changing surgery may have been especially vulnerable to the automatic reaction that dictates "discomfort means it's time to eat something." If you've done this several times a day for a decade or more, it stands to reason that this pattern has become ingrained in your thinking and behavior. For you, even more than for the average "dieter," it is vital that you let go of this pattern. One good binge after WLS surgery could send you to the hospital. I've seen it happen. Ruptured staples, blockages, or leaks can land you in ICU for months.

How do we "let go" of our love/hate relationship with eating for comfort? We do it a little at a time. If you've used food to cope for many years, you may not believe that you can move beyond this pattern. But let me reassure you that every time you let go of using food, there are a variety of fun, nurturing, and satisfying things to put in its place.

Anita Johnston, in her excellent book *Eating in the Light of the Moon*, uses this analogy: Imagine you have fallen into a raging river. In your efforts to keep from drowning, you grab onto a log. Initially, this decision saves your life, because clinging to the log allows you to keep your head above water and avoid drowning. But after a while, as the river carries you downstream into calmer waters, the log becomes a problem. Now clinging to it is the very thing that's holding you back! You can see the riverbank in the distance, and if you let go of the log, perhaps you can make it to shore. But the shore still seems a long way off, and you aren't sure you are a strong enough swimmer to get there. What if you started to swim to shore but couldn't make it? There are people on the shore calling, "Let go of the log!" Yet still you hesitate. How do you get out of this dilemma?

First, you let go of the log for just a few seconds at a time. You practice floating, then treading water, and when you get scared or tired you grab the log again and rest. Then you practice swimming around the log, first a few times, then many times as your strength and confidence grow. You swim a little ways toward the shore, then back to the log. Then you swim a little farther. Finally you are able to let go of the log entirely and swim to shore.

Every diet we've ever tried, every well-meaning but clueless person who has told us, "Quit overeating right now and get a grip on yourself," has ignored or misunderstood the reality of the log and the flooding river. We did, too. We bought into the idea that if we couldn't make this change all at once then we were flawed and defective in some important way. The following concept may help you realize that the opposite is true.

Honoring Your Resistance

Most of us have had moments (or, if you're like me, years) when we rebelled against the idea of a food plan or exercise. If our resistance— the part of us that can't or won't follow a food plan—is very strong, our initial reaction may be to criticize ourselves about it. We may feel ashamed and frustrated as we wonder, "What the #*&%@!! is wrong with me? I can do everything else in my life well, so why can't I seem to stick to a diet?"

There is another way to look at this dilemma, but be warned—it is a radical shift from how you may have viewed it in the past. Let's return to the drowning person holding onto the log.

If we can understand and have some compassion for the person who's scared to let go of the log, perhaps we can give that same part of ourselves permission to make changes in little steps, to learn to swim one stroke at a time. In doing so, we learn that it's okay to make our changes in a loving way rather than in the boot-camp drill-sergeant way. Has being strict or mean to yourself ever brought about positive, lasting change? I doubt it. Has demanding of yourself that you make a drastic change RIGHT NOW OR ELSE ever really worked? Not when part of you still resists doing it!

Instead, consider this: What if *nothing* is wrong with you? What if your resistance is actually there for a *good* reason? What if, instead of shaming and blaming yourself, you began to tell yourself, "All of my feelings deserve to be honored—even my resistance. Every feeling I experience has an important lesson to teach me. So right now, I'll slow down for a minute, breathe, and go within to discover what's going on."

One way of doing this could be to sit down with your journal and write out a "conversation" with your resistance—or with any feeling. You could write, "Resistance, I feel you wanting to rebel against this food plan. I feel you wanting to eat whatever you feel like eating, and the idea of being restricted is making you want to eat more! Yet I know there is more to this than needing food, because most of the time my body already feels full. So I want to ask you, resistance, what are you *really* trying to tell me?"

Then stay quiet for a minute or two, and write down whatever comes up from that resistant part of yourself. Continue asking and answering on paper until you feel finished. You may be surprised by what comes out. One thing is for sure: It will be about more than just food!

Cross-Addiction

Have you ever known someone who has successfully gotten rid of one bad habit only to pick up another? A common example is someone who gives up smoking but then gains twenty pounds. If you were to ask them about it they might say, "I can't help it; I have an addictive personality." Maybe you'd think, "Well that's just a stupid excuse, a cop-out." But what if there is some truth to that idea?

The fact is, cross-addiction—the tendency to become psychologically and/or physically dependent on a new behavior (like shopping or sex) or substance (like coffee or "energy" drinks) after having kicked another addiction—is very, very common. For those of us who have spent many years coping with life by using food, simply experiencing our feelings without any buffer sometimes gets too painful or scary. So we pick up another habit and fall right back into the pattern of coping with stress by using the new "fix" to soften life's sharp edges. Often without even realizing it, we come to depend on our new buffer more and more, until—guess what?—we are soon using it as much as we once used food!

Part of this behavior may be plain old bad habits—like going from enjoying one or two cups of coffee in the morning to having a whole pot. Or thinking you'll buy just one outfit for your new figure and ending up maxing out your credit card. One of the main signs of cross-addiction is this: We find something that gives us a feeling of pleasure or reward or comfort, and instead of using it just a little, we use it more and more—until it begins to damage the rest of our life in some way. Maybe it hurts us financially or harms our health. *But in spite of these problems, we keep doing it.* This is a hallmark of addiction, and it involves a cycle that progresses like this:

The Cycle of Addiction

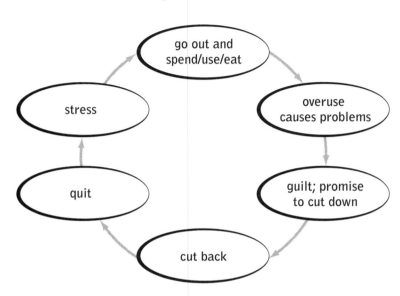

1. You use food, drugs, sex, etc., to cope with a stressful situation. Maybe you go overboard and use a little too much, or use "it" in a way you know isn't healthy for you.
2. When you go overboard, something bad happens.
3. Then you feel guilty and upset about the problem.
4. So you promise to change, cut back, or quit using.
5. You keep your promise for an hour, a day, a week—as long as you're still upset by the problem at hand.
6. But after things settle down, you forget your promise and why it was so important to quit.
7. Then the stresses of life happen, and pretty soon you start daydreaming of "it" and how it would make you feel better, help you cope, taste good, whatever.
8. The stress and the cravings both increase until you either get help or give in to the craving and relapse.

◎ Max's Story

Max is a forty-two-year-old delivery driver and father of three girls. He had WLS, dropped all his excess weight in the first year, and began going to the gym three times a week, where he lifted weights and walked on the treadmill. He began to feel really positive about his new body and the compliments he was receiving.

To look and feel even better, he started going to the gym every day after work. He also increased the length of his workout time, from 45 minutes, to 90 minutes, to spending 2–3 hours at the gym each evening. After a few months Max looked and felt pretty good. But he noticed that whenever he missed an exercise session, he became depressed or irritable. His wife and children were starting to complain that he never spent any time with them.

One evening, his youngest daughter's piano recital happened to coincide with his scheduled workout time. He promised to attend the recital, but then he made excuses, saying he had to stay late at work. In fact, he went to the gym rather than the recital. When his wife drove by the gym on the way home and spotted his car, he was caught, and they had quite a fight. His wife yelled and his daughter was in tears, but Max defended his actions—until his daughter shouted, "You don't love us anymore! All you love is your stupid exercise!" and ran to her room, crying.

Max said, "It was then that I understood not only was I being selfish, but I was also really damaging the very thing I loved most, my family. Why didn't I realize it sooner? I guess because the good feelings from the exercise—the endorphins—got me hooked just like the food had. So I cut back to going to the gym only three times a week again, and that has worked out okay."

Other Sources of Help

Sometimes we need more help than can be found in a book (even a fabulous book like this one) or from our friends. If we have tried everything we can think of and we're still getting nowhere—if we're at our wit's end—maybe what we need is to seek a different kind of help, such as specific treatment for eating-disorder issues.

Many of us believed that weight loss surgery was going to be the final answer and were disappointed to discover that eventually we could once again eat enough food to gain weight. Even now, at several years post-op, I can still become obsessed with food, still binge to some extent, and still gain weight. Living through a few episodes of this pattern has made me realize that if I'm not careful, I could become another gastric bypass failure statistic.

If you have tried everything, including the surgery; if it's appropriate for you, and you find yourself still overeating, still obsessed with food, and still riding the binge/diet cycle, you may want to consider treatment. Asking for this kind of help is nothing to be ashamed of. It doesn't mean anything bad about a person; in fact, it takes a great deal of honesty and courage to go after the kind of help you really need when nothing else is working. I've been a treatment counselor for thirteen years, but if I needed to, if I got so far into the obsessive/compulsive cycle again that I couldn't get out, I'd definitely seek treatment. There's a saying: "You can't save your face and your pride at the same time." If I had to choose, my pride would go out the window in favor of my health.

There are several kinds of treatment for addiction, each designed to provide a different level of care according to a person's individual needs. The following is an overview of the most common types:

Twelve-step groups and programs: Beginning with Alcoholics Anonymous, which was founded as a self-help group in 1935 to provide a supportive environment for recovery from alcoholism, the twelve-step philosophy has blossomed into hundreds of offshoot groups with millions of members worldwide. Some of these programs have to do with recovery from food addiction, such as Overeaters Anonymous, Compulsive Overeaters Anonymous, and Food Addicts Anonymous.

These groups are called "self-help" because they are free of charge and are run by their members. No specific length of treatment is recommended in twelve-step programs; they are considered to be lifelong programs as needed, like going to church or to the gym. Most twelve-step members report positive results from attending a few one-hour meetings per week and working with a "sponsor." A sponsor is a fellow group member who functions as a teacher/mentor and guides the newcomer through the twelve-step program of recovery. Once a person has completed the twelve steps and has remained abstinent for a period of time, he or she can sponsor other newcomers, and thus the program is kept alive.

Individual counseling: This involves meeting one-on-one with a counselor or therapist, hopefully one who is licensed and who has a lot of experience treating clients with issues similar to yours. These sessions usually last for an hour, and they can be scheduled once a week to once a month, depending on your needs. If you have medical insurance, it will usually cover twelve to twenty-four sessions of counseling per year. The benefit of this form of treatment is that it's totally geared to you and your needs. The drawback is that it lacks the component of group support, which can be especially helpful with eating-disorder issues.

Outpatient treatment: Outpatient treatment has three primary components: first, skill-building/education, in which you learn skills similar to those presented in this book. Second, group therapy, in which you join a group of people dealing with the same kinds of problems you have and talk things out in a safe, confidential group setting, facilitated by a trained therapist. Third, individual counseling and case management, which involves personal attention to your specific concerns. Typically, this sort of treatment program involves three-hour sessions occurring three times a week for eight to twelve weeks, but it could be shorter or longer depending on individual needs. Medical insurance usually covers outpatient treatment.

Residential treatment: This is live-in, twenty-four-hour-a-day treatment. You are fed, housed, and given a therapeutic daily schedule that involves education, skill-building, group counseling, individual counseling, exercise, meditation, and more. A case manager will be assigned to you and will make a customized list of your personal problems and goals called a "treatment plan." He or she will encourage and support you in meeting a series of small goals that will lead you into recovery, health, and wellness. The benefit of this kind of treatment is that it's a crash course in looking inward at yourself and in living a healthy lifestyle. The drawback is that you are in a "recovery cocoon" of sorts, insulated from the stresses and temptations of "real life."

Any one of these types of support, from the "as-needed" approach of twelve-step groups to the intensive work done in residential treatment, can be very helpful. Please don't be afraid or embarrassed to seek help if the methods you've been trying aren't working out.

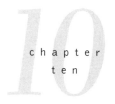

Love
and Intimacy
after
Losing the Weight

*Open your heart
without opening
the refrigerator*

I remember the first time I went clothes shopping after losing a hundred pounds. I walked into the store, looked around at the displays of current fashions—and just stood there. Where was I supposed to start? Although I knew shopping ought to be fun, my insides were in turmoil, having a confused conversation of their own. It went like this:

Come on, we've got to start somewhere. How about pants?

Fat girls don't wear pants. They show too much hips and thighs. Better look at long skirts.

But wait—I'm not fat anymore. My thighs don't even rub together!

Hmmm. Let's try some dresses. Long ones.

Why long ones? I'm sick of big stuff! Why can't I try a miniskirt?

A miniskirt—are you nuts? A nice, sensible dress is what we need.

Well, then, what kind of dress? Tropical? Professional? Miss Mary Anne?

Uhhhh, I don't know.

I don't know who I'm supposed to be anymore.

I knew the rules for dressing as a fat person. They were pretty simple. Depressing, but simple: Always wear loose-fitting, dark, sacklike things—nothing to draw attention to yourself or, God forbid, show your figure. Always wear high-heeled shoes, due to the mathematical theorem that a tall mass looks skinnier than a short one.

From my earliest years, I became skilled at fat couture—the many versions of the big dress, the big skirt, the pretty earrings to focus attention from the neck up. But I didn't need fat couture now. I had hundreds of options instead of just a few. In the fat-girl sizes, there had been only a handful of styles, none of them very attractive. But as a size six, all the pretty-girl fashions were available to me.

So that's great, right? Clothes shopping finally gets to be fun, instead of torture. This should be a cause for celebration, shouldn't it? And it was... except I had no clue what I was supposed to look like, no idea what "image" I wanted to present, in public or in private. Should I look sporty or flirty? Sweet or sultry? Artsy or professional? I really had no idea.

I tried on a few things and bought a few things. At first, they tended to be more form-fitting than before, a little shorter than before, a lot more youthful then before. Why? Because I could, damn it!

In the beginning it was a lot of fun wearing my new clothes. They made me feel young and free, like I'd never felt in my life. My first short skirt at age forty! Who knew? It was a heady experience—until I realized I was getting a little too much attention from the guys, and a few raised eyebrows from the women. So I selected looser clothes and buttoned them up a little more, and that felt better. I still looked nice, just not quite like Barbie. It took a while to figure out which clothes felt right for me. And as far as I could tell, the only way to find out was to try a few styles, until I found what fit—not just my figure, but my personality and my own sense of style.

Why am I going on about clothes shopping when this is a chapter about love?

Because my love life went the same way as my fashion life.

I didn't know what I wanted. Or rather, I knew I wanted true love, but I didn't know how to find it. After my ups and downs with Eric, I was a little gun-shy. I asked some friends for advice, and all of them said, "Make a list of what you want in a man." A list? Trying to be helpful, each friend offered a few of the qualities *they* thought a good partner should have. Pretty soon I had a list a mile long: smart, honest, handsome, funny, sweet, kind, upwardly mobile, rides motorcycles, likes to travel.... And on and on. Was there such a guy? And if there were, would he want me?

Again, I had no idea. I bounced back and forth from thinking I was a great catch and he'd be lucky to have me, to thinking I was the lowest creature on the planet, too old, too saggy, too whatever. Back and forth. And since I had no clue, it was easier to focus on the exterior qualities—on how I looked, how the guy looked, on the job, the car, the goals. So I spent the first couple of years after my bodily transformation going out with cute, young guys who were fun, adventurous, sometimes wealthy—guys who looked good on the outside, but still had some work to do on the inside, basically concerning how they handled their emotions and how they treated me. I spent a few months with one man and nearly a year with another, always looking for my "soul mate," as so many of us do. I never realized that maybe I was looking at the wrong things.

And, as was the case when shopping for clothes, I still had a bad case of "fat head" when it came to relationships. The typical fat-girl credo for a relationship is: *Oh thank God, someone loves me. Better hold on for dear life, because maybe no one else will.* Needless to say, this way of thinking wasn't very helpful.

Shopping for Mr. Right

Recently, a friend lured me to an Edward Jones investment seminar with the promise of a lobster lunch. As predicted, the food was better than the presentation, but one concept did stand out from the jargon about stocks, rates, and numbers. It was a good parable for the subject of love, so I'll share it with you.

The speaker, who was introduced as one of Edward Jones' top research analysts from New York, explained the firm's philosophy this way: "We at Edward Jones believe in three things—our 'commandments,' if you will. First, research your investments carefully, before you choose which one to buy. Second, make a quality choice, and, third, once you've chosen, hold on. Our experience shows that a quality choice will always increase its value over time."

Since I'd been thinking about relationships, I couldn't help but relate her comments to the subject of love as well as mutual funds. Whether you're building an investment portfolio or searching for a partner, these three things hold true. Here they are again:

Research your choice carefully. Know what you really want, and know what it's going to take to get it. Do you just want to have fun dating or do you want to settle down? What qualities are most important to you in a partner? Do you have those qualities yourself? What are your most cherished values? Like my friends said, it's helpful to make a list (see the assignments below). When doing so, be sure to identify a few qualities that are your nonnegotiables (like honesty, kindness, perhaps earning a decent living), and realize that some qualities, while desirable (like wearing Italian shoes or loving your favorite TV show), really aren't that big a deal.

Make a quality choice. *Believe that you are worth loving, and that you are worthy of living your dreams.* Don't let the ex–fat person in your head run your love life! You have lots of choices today. It's a delicate balance: You don't want to be too perfectionistic or picky, but nor do you want to merely settle. When Goldilocks went into the bear's cottage, everything she found at first—the porridge, the beds—was either too hot or too cold, too hard or too soft. She had to hold out for the one that was just right, and she did. So do you. Make a quality choice.

Once you've chosen, hold on for the long term. In our instant-gratification society, it's far too easy to drop something—or someone—once the going gets tough. But if you want a genuine partnership, guess what? The going *will* get tough at times. It pays to stick around long enough to see how things play out with someone you really care about, rather than hopping from one infatuation to another.

I don't mean you should hang in there if your gut is telling you it's not a good fit, and I'm certainly not suggesting that you stick around for any abuse, not at all, but—here's a reality check. After about six months of dating, once both partners' best behavior wears off, your issues are going to bump up against the other person's issues, and there will be some friction, some conflict, some negotiation. If you work through this stuff, and with a bit of luck, you'll end up with increased understanding and a deepening of your love.

So, what do you really want in an intimate relationship? A quick à la carte snack or the full entrée? If you haven't had much experience in relationships, perhaps you'll want to take some time and just date around so you can learn about yourself and what you want in a partner. I'm not suggesting that you *sleep* around; just enjoy some coffee or dinner dates. Taste a few "snacks" without creating a lot of pressure or worries about the future. Lots of folks do this; that's why it's called dating!

On the other hand, if you've already had enough "practice" with relationships and you're ready for the entrée, perhaps it's time to make a quality choice and stay with it.

Remember what our Edward Jones guru said: "A quality investment always increases its value over the long term." Who am I to argue with Wall Street?

◎ Margie's Story

Margie is a forty-five-year-old warehouse manager whom I met while I was waiting to have WLS. Even though we're the same age, our lives have been very different. Whereas I've had a series of relationships and have been married, she hasn't. By age forty, she had never even been on a date. Like most of her family members, she'd been obese since childhood. Consequently, she'd never had any experience with men.

That's not to say she didn't have a full life. Although Margie had weighed over 350 pounds for most of her adult life, she excelled in her work and enjoyed an active social life with her friends. She was smart, witty, and had a great sense of humor. But in terms of romantic relationships, she was still like a child: innocent, hopeful, and naive.

Then she had weight loss surgery, dropped over two hundred pounds, and ventured into the social scene, where her dating situation changed almost overnight. On Saturday nights she'd go to a dance club, and soon she learned how to mix, mingle, and dance sexy. She was having fun and enjoying her new figure and self-confidence. It wasn't long before Margie began dating her first boyfriend, and, a few months later, her second, both of whom she met on the dance floor.

On the surface Margie was handling all of this just fine, but underneath, she confessed to me, she felt like she was navigating her way through the Amazon jungle without a map.

For all of us who, like Margie, are trying to steer our way through the wonderfully confusing world of relationships, a couple of assignments are presented below. They're designed to help you get clear on where you stand and where you're going.

ASSIGNMENT: The List for Dating

You've got it, we're going to make a list, just like my friends suggested. If you are in the "just dating" phase of relationships, your list should begin with the very basics. If you're unsure of the answers to some of the following questions, ask people you trust how they would respond (but not how *you* should respond; that's up to you.) If you decide to read up on the subject, be warned: There are a bazillion books out there on how to date, who to date, and how to act on a date. There's even a book called *The List*. But don't worry. I'll give you the cheat sheet on what they all have to say.

The common themes found in dating books are as follows:

First and most important, ***respect and love yourself.*** Be the best you can be, and you will attract a partner who does the same.

Second, *be yourself.* Be sincere, be for real. Don't feel you need to turn yourself inside out to keep a partner happy. If that's what the situation requires, it's probably not a good fit. Besides, being true to yourself and your values will save you a lot of time. You'll weed out the junk dates and attract those who speak your language.

Third, *keep on being yourself no matter what.* Hold on to all the things that make you you. If you always go to church or the gym, don't stop because your date thinks it's silly. If you like old movies and your date doesn't, keep watching them. Just go with a friend who likes them too. Ultimately, what will work best when you're dating is what feels right to you in your heart, mind, and spirit. And if you keep up with all the friends, hobbies, and healthy habits you had when you first met your love interest, you'll continue being an interesting, vital person who's fun to date, and you'll be too busy to be taken for granted!

Last, *if love is what you want, give it generously, and open your heart to receive it fully.* Yes, I know we need to be careful in today's world. Nobody wants to be manipulated or hurt. But sometimes, perhaps because of a painful past history or because we're just too scared to open up to love, we let a situation that *could* bloom into a beautiful romance wither and die from lack of nourishment. If you really want it, you've got to step up to the plate and go for it!

Okay, end of sermon. Back to the assignment.

Answer these questions in your journal:

1. What are my values (e.g., honesty, integrity, kindness, financial security, emotional security, strength of character, generosity)?

2. Which of the above values matter most to me? (List your top three.)

3. What is important to me in a relationship—emotional support, lots of affection, fun adventures, similar religion or politics, someone who takes care of me, someone who is very attractive? Some of your answers may repeat things you listed in items 1 and 2.

4. Which of the things I named in item 3 are most important to me? (List three.)

5. How do I want to be treated by a date? For example, do I want to plan ahead or be spontaneous? Do I want someone who's always on time, or is it okay if they tend to be late? Who pays? Who decides where to go?

6. How will I know if it's a good fit and I want to get closer to the person?

7. How will I know if it's not a good fit and I want out? What do I say if the time comes to end things?

8. Is there someone supportive I can talk to about my dating adventures? Someone I trust and who will help me gain perspective and balance? If not, where can I find someone like this?

Those of you who are only interested in casual dating can stop here. Those of you who want a quality partnership can complete the following assignment, too.

ASSIGNMENT: The List for a Relationship

In your journal, write at the top of a page, "What I'd Like in a Partner." Divide the page in half vertically, and label one side "Inside Qualities" and the other "Outside Qualities."

1. As you did when compiling your list for dating, think about your values. Which of these are most important to you in a long-term partner? List these under "Inside Qualities."

2. Also under "Inside Qualities," list personality and character traits you'd like in a partner, such as intelligence, sense of humor, helpfulness, kindness, a giving nature, morality, truthfulness, etc. (There may be some overlap between this list and the list of values you compiled.) Do you want a partner who is spiritually focused or not? Responsible or not? How important to you is that "spark" of romantic attraction? Do you want lots of affection and romance, or is that less important to you compared to other things?

3. Under "Outside Qualities," list the more material and worldly things you'd like to have in a partner. For example, do you care what kind of job or income they have? Do you want a partner to be goal-oriented? If so, what sorts of goals are important to you? Do you want your partner to go to church? Is it important to you that a potential partner would want kids? What if they already have kids? Is it okay if they smoke? Drink? Live like a slob or are neat as a pin? Is your ideal partner more traditional in their view of gender roles, or more modern? More carefree or more ambitious? Do they dress fancy or casual? What activities do they like? What skills do they have? How much education?

   Write down as many qualities on both sides of the page as you can think of. For now, don't worry about how many you've listed or how important each one is. Just get them down on paper.

4. Once you have made both lists as complete as you can, number each quality in each list in order of priority. In other words, looking at your "Inside Qualities" list, which ones do you feel are absolutely essential, and which would be nice but are optional? Make the most important number one, the next most important number two, and so on. Then do the same thing for the "Outside Qualities" list.

Congratulations! You have now created an absolutely wonderful, if unreal, partner. The reason I've asked you to number your desired qualities in order of their importance is because you probably won't get them all in a single person. Not because you don't deserve them, but because nobody is perfect. I'm certainly not—are you? Then how can we expect perfection in a potential partner? For this reason, it helps to be clear on what is *most* important to you in a loving partnership, on what really matters over the long term.

Until you find that not-quite-perfect (but just right for you) someone, I suggest you emphasize and enjoy all aspects of your single life—your friendships, personal goals, family relationships, and hobbies.

Not only will doing so help you fend off any feelings of loneliness; it will help you be a healthier, happier, more interesting person when you do start a new relationship, or when you revitalize the one you've got.

Speaking of which...

If You're Already in a Relationship

◉

During my career as an addictions counselor I've often worked with my clients' spouses and family members to help them create a supportive environment at home. Loved ones of people in recovery are often closely involved in the recovery process. In this context, therefore, "relationship" means anything from your intimate partnership, to your family relationships, to any other connection that's significant enough to have the potential to either strengthen or sabotage your recovery.

Relationships have a life of their own. They have patterns, rhythms, currents, and undercurrents. When one person starts making changes, even positive ones, those familiar rhythms get disrupted. On the surface, everyone wants the addict—whether a drug addict or a food addict—to get healthy and stay that way. But adjusting to change isn't easy for anyone, because change can bring up uncomfortable emotions.

This is where the recovery process for the food addict and the drug addict are *not* the same. Alcohol and drug addicts tend to create havoc for themselves and everyone around them. Their loved ones are kept busy taking care of them, covering up for them, and cleaning up the messes they make. With compulsive overeaters, it is usually the exact opposite. They themselves are usually the caretakers, doing all the cooking, cleaning, and breadwinning for their families, nurturing everyone but themselves, then turning to food for their own nurturing and comfort.

After WLS, this has to change if the post-op patient is to receive the care they need. They will need to allow loved ones to take over some of the household responsibilities, not only while they are recovering from surgery, but thereafter. This may create problems; family members who are used to having everything done for them may resent having to take up the slack. Talking about these issues prior to surgery often produces good results, as does deciding how everything from chores to conflict resolution will be handled. A good WLS program offers counseling for both the patients and their families.

Other common relationship issues for WLS patients are those of compatibility, communication, and changes in status and power as the patient loses weight and becomes more attractive. Many of my clients have brought up the issue of wanting to "upgrade" how they are treated in relationships. When we're big, we feel bad about ourselves, and this is reflected in society—in how we're treated by teachers, employers, even our families. We may end up staying in situations, jobs, or relationships that aren't good for us. But as we lose the weight and become healthier and more confident, we may find the courage to make changes that will help us keep growing and becoming the happy, contented people we were meant to be. Below, Helen talks about the evolution in her marriage that took place after she underwent weight loss surgery.

◎ Helen's Story

"I met my husband, Brad, when we were both in our thirties. We worked together in a downtown café where I was a waitress and he was a bartender. I was self-conscious about being overweight, but he didn't seem to mind. We fell in love, got married, and had two kids in three years. Everything was great, except that with each baby I gained more weight, until by the time our youngest was four, I was nearing 250 pounds.

"Sometimes Brad would comment on my weight, although he was never really mean about it. But when the doctor said I was developing high cholesterol and high blood pressure and was at risk for heart disease, we agreed it was time to do something.

"I tried to diet, but I had a really hard time with it. Brad and the kids were used to my cooking big hearty meals for them that were full of all the yummy things I was supposed to stop eating myself. I couldn't seem to make them understand how hard it was for me to have all those sweets and starches right under my nose yet not eat them! 'Just use your willpower,' Brad would say, or, 'Just have one bite, and leave the rest.' I knew he was right, and I felt even worse about myself because I wasn't able to do that. I was getting nowhere, and we were fighting more than we ever had over my eating and my weight.

"By the time I decided to have the surgery, we were both tired of fighting and eager for a solution, so we had very few conflicts over it. After the surgery, Brad was really good about taking care of me, and at first our family got the message—'Mommy's 'sick,' so we have to take care of her.' I have to say, after I'd spent the past several years being—well, being Mommy—it was really nice to let somebody take care of me for a change. I used a treadmill for exercise every day, and they kept the junk food hidden away where I didn't have to see it.

"We started to have problems again around my tenth month post-op. By then I'd lost about ninety-five pounds and was feeling better than I had in years. I was feeling so good, so much more confident and positive about myself, about my health, how I looked, about the future—everything. All of a sudden I had a lot of positive energy. I talked to Brad about starting my own business or going back to work outside the home. That's when all hell broke loose.

"He became really resentful and sarcastic. He'd say, 'You just want to go out and show off how you look now; you're so full of yourself,' and other comments along those lines. He started bringing home lots of junk food and candy again, even though we'd agreed

(cont'd.)

to keep that stuff to a minimum. I became resentful, too. Was this the man I'd married? Why was he trying to sabotage me? Didn't he want me to succeed?

"These were some really disturbing things for me to consider, and hurtful, too. Rather than face these issues head on, I found myself giving up. I figured, 'What's the use?' and went back to eating the junk food that was all over our house again. Before I knew it, I'd gained fifteen pounds. When I finally realized that the surgery wasn't going to protect me anymore from gaining weight, I really got scared. I asked Brad if we could go back into counseling, and at first he said he was too busy. So I went by myself.

"The counselor helped me to understand what was happening. He helped me see that, instead of facing the problems in my marriage, or what might happen if I was to nurture my own potential, I'd gone back to hiding behind food. I'd gone back to being 'the weak one'—and I was on my way back to being 'the fat one' if I didn't turn things around somehow.

"I decided that if I kept on this way with my eating, I would end up hating myself. Even if my marriage stayed intact, the cost—my healthy new self—was too high. So I took some action.

"I sat my family down for a talk. I explained to them that, just like a disease, my overeating was a danger to my health and I needed their help. At the counselor's advice, I didn't blame or sermonize. I just kept repeating, 'This is a serious health problem for me, and I really need your help.' When they asked what kind of help, I asked them to please go back to hiding the junk food from Mommy. For the kids this was like a game, so they agreed.

"With Brad, it took a little more time. I told him I loved him and wanted our marriage to work, but I needed some kind of a personal life, too. I told him I intended to go back to work, and that along with work I'd try my best to fulfill what the family needed. And I encouraged him to join me in counseling whenever he was willing.

"For another week or two he kept up the pressure on me to stay home—or, really, to stay my old codependent self! The cookies and candy were still on the kitchen countertops, but I didn't bite the bait. I just kept putting the junk food away in the boys' bedroom and kept going on job interviews until I found a job I liked.

"Now I've been working at a women's gym for the past two months, and I love it. It has really helped me get back on track with my exercise and eating, too. Once my husband realized that I was going to do whatever it took to keep my health and my life on track, he backed off and accepted my new job. Just last week he even apologized for making such a big deal out of it! I'm glad I stuck to my guns and didn't back down, or who knows where we'd be today?"

Whatever your relationship situation, dear reader, don't lose hope. Find and utilize a support system, like Helen did with her counselor, and most of all, don't give up.

It *is* possible to have the kind of love that brings joy and deep satisfaction into your heart and soul. It you want it, seek kindly and gently until it finds you. There is an old saying: "If I keep a green branch in my heart, the singing bird will come." It will.

And if you're already in a loving partnership, for heaven's sake, don't take it for granted! Show your beloved your appreciation as often as you can. It's the only thing that really matters.

Maintenance
Enjoying the Banquet
of a Gourmet Life

Before enlightenment,
chop wood, carry water.
After enlightenment,
chop wood, carry water.

— Zen saying

Imagine this happy future for yourself: You've succeeded! You've learned to eat well, you are enjoying exercise, and—wonder of wonders—you have even dropped the weight you wanted to lose. You have learned to make self-nurturing choices in all areas of your life, and you're getting positive strokes and compliments from those around you. In short, everything is flowing along smoothly.

But once you get to where you want to go, and the compliments happen less frequently because you've looked good for a while, your new way of life may lose its spark of novelty and become humdrum. You'll get used to looking and feeling better, and all of the reasons why you "hit bottom" in the first place will start to fade from memory. You'll carry on, but maybe underneath the satisfaction of having achieved your goal you'll begin to wonder, "What am I supposed to do with the rest of my life?" All the time and energy you used to put into dieting, eating, thinking about dieting, thinking about eating, feeling guilty when you've overeaten, feeling hopeful when you've found a new miracle diet—all that energy is freed up now, for you to do...what? What will you do with the time and energy that you've worked so hard to gain?

Well, what do the "civilians" do? They live their lives. Ideally, they have meaningful relationships, do productive work, and have an enjoyable social life. They feel a part of their community, live in accordance with their values, and have some way in which they give back to their families, friends, or community. Maybe they have satisfying hobbies or interests, something they feel passionate about, and a way to play.

When you enter the maintenance phase of this program, it will be important to continue to pay attention to your choices and to continue following your nutrition and exercise plan. You may decide to amend your plan from time to time to meet your changing needs, and certainly your food choices will broaden as time passes after your weight loss surgery. I've amended my food plan several times, sometimes to eliminate more binge foods and sometimes to add nutritional supplements, like a daily "green drink" made of spirulina and barley greens, which help to detoxify and alkalize the body. Nowadays I do more strength training than aerobic exercise, although I still love my hikes. We aren't static; we grow and change, and we must find ways to adapt without moving too far away from the foundation that brought us this far.

Get Busy Doing What You Love and You'll Forget to Eat

◎

More than just our food plan may need to be modified over time. The goal is to create a life that feels happy, satisfying, and full without being overwhelming. Many of us have used food to mask the troublesome question, "What do I want to be when I grow up?" I know some folks who are still asking this question at age thirty-five, forty, or even older. The days when people worked at one job for their whole lives and then retired with a pension seem to be over. I've heard a statistic that most folks who work for a living will typically change careers at least three times.

If you are not enjoying the part of your life that includes work, career, or avocation, then by all means do something about it. If you spend a forty-hour week doing something that rubs you the wrong way, you're sacrificing a lot of precious time to feeling discontented. I don't know about you, but for me, feeling uncomfortable for a long-enough period will definitely make me want to eat.

The good news is that the reverse is also true. When I'm doing something I really enjoy, something that makes my soul happy and my spirit sing, *I forget to eat.* Believe me, this is really a miracle for a compulsive eater. Have you ever met a perpetually slim person who, when they encounter a problem, says, "Oh, I just can't eat, I'm too upset"? Please. For thirty years of my life, there was no such thing as being "too upset" to eat. When you were upset, you ate twice as much! I have eaten my way through breakups, makeups, hissy fits, sicknesses, and deaths. I have used food, both unconsciously and consciously, to numb painful feelings on many, many occasions.

Yet when I am working on a painting, or decorating a house, or writing, I feel excited, satisfied, and fully engaged in my project. Several hours can pass in this pleasant, happily occupied state of mind, until actual physical hunger or some other commitment tears me away. When I'm involved in a project I love, there's no such thing as being bored. I take my folder of drawings and other projects with me everywhere, and if I'm stuck with some time on my hands I'll pull them out and work on them. For example, right now, in addition to this book, I'm working on four other projects: two tattoo designs, a mandala painting for a friend's birthday, and perfecting my sugar-free, wheat-free oatmeal cookie recipe. (Yep, they're good!) These are fun, no-pressure projects, but that's not always the case. Last month, I entered a prestigious annual art contest, and I worked hard to get my piece just right for the show. All these projects, from the silly to the serious, are designed to keep my creative juices flowing, *and to give me something to do besides eating when I have extra time on my hands and I don't know what to do with it.*

I have one friend who's both a city bus driver and a classical pianist, and I have another who's an auto mechanic and creates beautiful stone waterfalls and does nature photography in his free time. Then there's my friend Lisa, who's an oil painter and a nature lover and who works as a landscape architect. She gets to apply all the things she loves to do to what she does for a living. I even know a few "purists"—people who only create art or music or poetry and who make a good living doing just that.

Maybe you have long held on to a cherished dream of pursuing your talents in art or music or something else, yet over the years this dream was buried by the daily grind of life's little responsibilities. Now is the perfect time to dust off your dream and see how it looks and feels. Is it still something you'd love to do? Or are there other interests that tug at your heart and make you think, "Gee, I'd like to try that, but..."? Now is the time to get rid of the "but"—literally and figuratively—and to find a way to make time for yourself and your heart's desires.

Maybe you have never felt very "artistic," and outside of your normal routine there isn't any hobby or creative project that you yearn to do. That's okay, too. It just means you have a wonderful opportunity to find out what you enjoy, to discover what's fun and interesting to you.

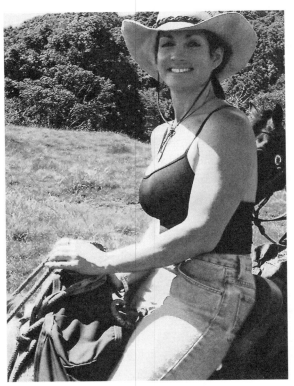

Horseback riding at Piiholo Ranch

One of my class members, Stella, had a pretty great life—so great, in fact, I found myself wondering why she was taking the class in the first place. She was maybe five pounds overweight, and she wasn't anorexic or bulimic. She had a good marriage, great kids, and a big house in the country with horses, dogs, and cats. Her only concern, she said, was that "after dinner when the kids are busy doing their homework, and there are no specific tasks left for the day, I find myself wandering around the house with nothing to do. I always seem to end up in the kitchen, nibbling on something like cookies or popcorn or a bag of chips. Then I take the food into the den and watch TV with my husband. And pretty soon I'll have eaten the whole bag without even realizing it. That's the kind of thing I want to stop doing."

The other class members came up with lots of potential solutions for her, some impractical, some funny, some useful. They suggested she do yoga stretches on the floor in front of the TV, watch an exercise video instead of TV, do a puzzle, have more sex, sew something, or make crafty projects as she watched TV. She chose to learn how to make beaded earrings, necklaces, and bracelets. She had so much fun making jewelry and giving it away that by the time the class ended she was thinking of selling it in local boutiques. And she enjoyed herself so much while she was involved in her creative endeavor that she forgot to eat!

◎ Elaine's Story

Elaine, a twenty-five-year-old college student, was about six months post-op when her appetite began to return with a vengeance. Although she'd already lost over fifty pounds, she had about a hundred more to go, and she was scared to death that the return of her urge to overeat meant that she wouldn't lose any more weight.

She discussed her predicament in her OEE class and began to address the cravings on several levels at once. At the physical level, she took special care with her diet, making sure to eat several small, protein-based meals throughout the day. To her regimen of daily vitamins she added the amino acid L-glutamine, which can help keep cravings at bay. To deal with the mental and emotional aspects of her urge to overeat, she committed to calling at least two friends every day to check in, and she also wrote in her journal each day.

(cont'd.)

Elaine also realized that she didn't have enough to do in the evenings, which was typically when her cravings were at their worst. Using the methods described in the following handout, she identified three things she enjoyed doing but hadn't done in a long time — sewing, dancing, and ceramics. The most practical one to do in the evenings at home was sewing, so she pulled out her sewing machine and began to make clothes. As her weight continued to drop, she altered some of her favorite outfits, trimming them down to fit her shrinking figure. By the last class session, Elaine felt that she had passed over this hurdle. She said, "I feel like I've gotten into a new groove. Instead of snacking, I'm doing something productive that I enjoy."

With these ideas in mind, let's take a look at the following assignment.

ASSIGNMENT: Identifying My Likes and Dislikes

Write your answers to the following questions in your journal. Where I've asked you to list "four things" or "three things," etc., feel free to add as many more options as you like.

1. Write down four things you really enjoy doing.
2. Write down three things you would really like to learn how to do (or to do better).
3. If money, time, and freedom were abundant, what would you love to be doing?
4. Write down two things you do regularly that take up too much of your time.
5. With the two things from #4 in mind, what are some ways you could set boundaries to give yourself some free time?
6. When you take good care of yourself physically, mentally, and emotionally, how do you feel?

7. When you neglect yourself physically, mentally, or emotionally, how do you feel?

8. Looking at your answers to the last two questions, how important is it to make time to nurture yourself?

ASSIGNMENT: Commit to Enjoying Yourself

After completing the above assignment, now identify a specific time of day when you usually want to overeat, and come up with three activities you can do instead. Be proactive. Don't wait for the cravings to hit; get busy doing what you love and you'll forget all about them! Here's an example: After 7 p.m., when I usually want to snack, instead I will—

o drink a cup of tea and read a good book

o do a sewing or craft project

o call a friend

o check out the extensive list on pages 229–230 for more ideas

Spiritual Vitamins

I'm so grateful for my weight loss surgery, and for learning about the tools that have kept me on track. And so far, the process has been a success. Over the first year post-op, I lost 80 to 90 pounds, and over the second year I lost maybe 15 or 20 more. Yes, I've had my rough spots, and, yes, my weight has fluctuated 5 to 15 pounds over the past several years. But more important, I've stuck to my new routines, which have allowed me to stay at a reasonable weight (135 to 145 pounds, give or take a little).

At times I've struggled to stay focused on exercising, eating right, and all the other aspects of recovery that need regular attention. Distractions have occasionally lured me away from my healthy rituals for an hour or a day or a week—but generally never longer than that. I've gotten to the point where these rituals (I call them "rituals" because for some reason I still hate the word "discipline") feel really good to me. They feel centering, nourishing, and like they give me the strength to go through my day in the best possible way.

Here is my typical schedule: I get up around seven, have coffee, and say my prayers. On two or three mornings of the week I go to a twelve-step meeting. Next I go for an uphill hike with my dog in the forest. I consider my hike the most important part of my day, because it helps me stay physically, mentally, and spiritually fit. While I'm hiking, I pray out loud (there's nobody else around when I hike, in case you were wondering), thanking Spirit for everything I'm grateful for. I ask for God's help in my daily affairs, and I surrender the results to God's will. Then I attempt to be quiet, putting aside the relentless mental chatter in my head as best I can. After that I try simply to remain open, breathing the crisp morning air, listening to the distant birdsong, seeing the misty bands of sunlight filter down through the branches. It is so beautiful up there, on any day, in any kind of weather. Just being outside in nature nurtures the soul in a way I can't explain. Sometimes I'll take a friend along on these walks, and we enjoy a good heart-to-heart talk while we hike.

Back at home, I plan my food for the day, starting with a protein-based drink or meal and my vitamins, along with my breakfast. My workday goes from 10 or 11 A.M. till 5 or 6 P.M. Before I start working, I plan whatever else I need to do that day, making room for a balance of work time during the day and downtime in the evening. I make sure to have dinner before 8 P.M., and to set aside time, even if only a few minutes, for prayer and meditation before bed. I try to get to bed by 10:30 or 11. If I can't sleep, I'll get up, make a cup of soothing tea, write in my journal, then go back to bed by midnight at the latest; otherwise it's hard to get up.

My life sounds simple, but I have spent years perfecting my daily ritual through much trial and error. For example, I've found it's a good idea to plan your most energetic activities during the part of the day when you have the most energy. For me, that's the morning, so that's when I exercise and take care of personal business. If I try to squeeze in exercise later in the day, or put it off until the afternoon or evening, when I have less energy, more often than not I'll flake out and then feel guilty about it. But if I start my day with both a physical and spiritual grounding, it helps inspire me to make healthy choices throughout the rest of the day.

Do I do this perfectly every time? Of course not. Certain things are flexible, but my hike, my food plan, my prayers, and my meetings are not. I need these routines to be rock solid, because for many years before surgery I told myself, "Well, one day off from exercise won't hurt, right?" Or, "One piece of cake is no big deal." But you know what? It is a big deal. Every little choice I make either helps to establish patterns of recovery or drags me back into old behavior, which leads eventually to my gaining weight and feeling horrible about myself. Didn't I do that for enough years already?

A few years ago, my friend's son Travis, who was seven or eight at the time, would watch me leave for a twelve-step meeting right after breakfast every morning. Often he would ask, "Auntie, why do you go to those meetings every morning? What is it for? Is it like school?" I said, "Well, Trav, it is kind of like school. I go there to learn how to be healthy and how to be close to God—kind of like spiritual vitamins. You take a Flintstones vitamin every day so you won't get sick, right?" He nodded. I said, "It's kind of like that."

It's also like going to the gym. If I work out regularly, I'll get results, see positive changes, and feel good about myself. If I work out half-heartedly, I'll get halfhearted results. And when I look back on many of the behaviors that used to be comfortable to me—like being a slug, overeating, wishing for good changes to happen in my life but not doing anything about it—I see that slowly but surely they have become *un*comfortable.

The most important key to staying consistent with these maintenance activities is to find things you really enjoy doing and to do them often. My hike in the forest is one of my favorite things to do in the world. So of course I keep doing it! In that way, the very things I used to complain and procrastinate about—exercise, taking vitamins, sticking to some kind of a food plan—these things are becoming my comfort zone. Because when I do them, I feel energetic, positive, and self-confident. And when I don't, I don't.

As you can see, getting and staying healthy hasn't been a big, earth-shaking revelation from on high; instead, it has involved a million little daily choices—sometimes easy, sometimes challenging—that continue to move me forward in a positive direction.

Kind of like taking your vitamins.

"Dayenu"

Not long ago I attended a Passover seder with my friend Lisa. A seder is a six-thousand-year-old ceremony retelling the story of the exodus of the Jews from Egypt. It was a beautiful ritual, with lots of songs, prayers, candle lighting, and symbolic foods. Lisa likes anything "witchy," and she looked at me with raised eyebrows every time the ceremony resembled something pagan, which it often did.

The leader of the ceremony, Eve, introduced us to the Hebrew word *dayenu*. We even sang a song about it. According to Eve, *dayenu* means "it would have been enough, we would have been satisfied with just a little, but God gave us so much." She said the deeper meaning is to be grateful for all the little steps on the path of learning; don't just focus on the goal, but honor your progress for each accomplishment you make, however small. *Dayenu* is saying thank you for those steps, knowing that every one of them is necessary.

As the seder ended, I offered to help Eve with the dishes, and soon we were chatting pleasantly in the kitchen while we cleaned up. Eve is a doctor, and she has written a book called *Culinary Potions,* so I felt safe talking with her about some of my eating and nutritional concerns. I was about to start teaching another Overcoming Emotional Eating class the very next day, and as often happens on the night before a new class, I was having an attack of insecurity. I said to Eve, "I'm not sure if I'm the best teacher for this. After all, it's not like I'm a perfect example of proper eating behavior all the time. I could stand to lose another fifteen pounds, and I'm not doing very well at it right now. I mean, I'm doing okay—just not as well as I would like to be."

Eve smiled and said, "*Dayenu,* right? You've come a long way already, and you have all of that experience, strength, and hope to share. At the least, you probably know more than they do."

Now that was a way of looking at it that I hadn't even considered. I found myself explaining the concept of *dayenu* to the new class members the next day, and I've thought about it ever since. Honoring where we are right now and acknowledging the strengths and lessons we've gained through hard-won experience gives us the encouragement we need to take the next step. And the next one.

Dayenu.

A Final Thought

Another thing happened at the seder that made a big impression on me. After dinner, Eve's boyfriend, Greg, told us about not one but *two* major accidents and subsequent near-death experiences he had been through in the past five years. He said, "I know it sounds crazy, but those accidents turned out to be the best thing that ever happened to me. When I died, or almost died, I saw a lot of things most people don't get to see during their lives. I live with a real sense of peace now, because I saw where we came from, and I saw where we're going when we die."

He had us all spellbound. "So, where *are* we going?" one girl asked him. He laughed and said, "Not far, not far at all. I have this desire nowadays to go around telling everybody how much I love them, and to tell them that the most important thing we can do in this life is just to show love, to demonstrate love. It's actually very simple—that's all we're really here to do."

As I looked into his open, peaceful face, a lot of my illusions and preconceptions about life began to fall away. Could it really be that simple? Was this way of living—to show more love—really the answer? It certainly sounded right. And I was hearing it from the horse's mouth, so to speak. I believed that Greg had been where he said he'd been, and that what he was telling us was the truth.

I guess it's not about losing those last few pounds, or about making our goals happen, or even about improving our relationships. It's about bringing love into every situation, and showing love to others as best we can.

That's all we need to know, and all we need to do. Just show love.

I believe it.

I'm gonna do it.

How about you?

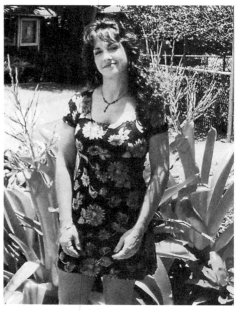

Over forty in a miniskirt. Who knew?

One final thought for you, dear reader: A common theme I notice with my clients is that we get so focused on the goals we're trying to achieve that *we forget to appreciate where we are*. It's wonderful to reach for the best self we can be, as long as we can love ourselves along the way. Lighten up, see the humor in things, and enjoy the heck out of *this* moment, right now. Why not?

Go on, I dare you.

Look around you, look inside yourself, and take this moment to deeply appreciate all the things that are going well in your life. Be grateful for everything that has brought you to this moment of clarity, this place of hope for your future, this step toward living your dreams. Be thankful for all the growth you've made so far.

And from that place of thankfulness, anything is possible.

All the best to you on your journey!

A Sample Plan:
Nurturing Foods, Movement Choices, and Fun Tools

Traditional weight loss programs have been divided into two camps. The most popular has been the body camp, which says, "Eat this, don't eat that, exercise your butt off, and, remember, no pain no gain!"—as if that's all you'll ever need. Sound familiar? Well, if that method really worked, then there would be only one diet, we'd all have done it perfectly the first time around, everyone would have kept the weight off once and for all—and that would be the end of it. Yet there are hundreds, maybe thousands, of diets out there, and let's face it: They *all* basically say, "Eat less, exercise more." Right? So why haven't we done it?

Then there's the psychology camp, which says, "If you'll just heal your mental and emotional problems, then the weight will fall away as if by magic." Magic? I used to believe in magic. Magic to me meant that if I were reading a self-help book while eating cookies, those calories didn't count. The psychological method did give me some insight into how and why I overate, but I was still overeating! The knowledge I'd gained about myself didn't seem to stop the cravings. I didn't understand how I could be so competent and accomplished in every other area of my life, yet continue overeating. It was frustrating and depressing, and at times I felt hopeless.

All that changed when I learned how to bring the two camps together, which is the strategy outlined in this book.

In this Appendix, I'll present a sample food plan. I encourage you *not* to follow it religiously! Instead, use it as a basic framework to help you develop your *own* plan, tailored to your body's needs. A cautionary note: If you have any health challenges or concerns, please get your doctor's feedback and support before putting any nutritional or supplement changes into action.

Let's start with a shopping list. Only go shopping when you're *not* hungry! You can use my list as a place to start and add to or subtract from it based on what works for you. What do I mean by "what works for you"? Foods that work for you will cause you to feel satisfied yet still energetic and clear-headed. Foods that aren't good for you will leave you feeling tired, sluggish, or foggy. They may produce gas, mucus, or let you know in other ways that your body is fighting to overcome their effects. Often, in spite of these ill effects, these foods will also generate cravings to keep you eating more of the same.

You may have to experiment to find what foods work for you and to determine what trigger foods you'll binge on no matter how healthy they seem. Once you have figured it out, stick to your list, and avoid the trap that says, "I'll just buy this treat for _____ because I know they'll really enjoy it." How many times did that treat end up being yours? Stick to your list.

Sample Shopping List
◎

Proteins

Beef	Chicken	Fish	Shellfish	Eggs
Tofu	Tempeh	Turkey	Lamb	Pork

Protein/carb combos

Beans: red, black, pink, white
Vegetable proteins such as TVP (textured vegetable protein)
Split peas
Hummus/garbanzo beans (chickpeas)
Lentils

Proteins plus healthy fats

Nuts
Peanut butter (no added sugar)

Dairy proteins

Milk	Cottage cheese	Yogurt
Cheese	Goat cheese	

Powdered/liquid proteins for protein drinks

Whey protein (if you are okay with dairy)
Soy protein drink powders (like Spiru-Tein, if you are okay with soy)
Liquid protein drinks such as Isopure, Myoplex, etc., as long as they are
    sugar free.

Liquid protein drinks can be found at GNC or similar stores. My favorites are the EAS Advantage Carb Control protein drinks because
they taste good, they are sugar free, and each serving contains 15 grams
of protein, only 100 calories, and lots of vitamins. EAS products are not
organic, but you can certainly make an organic protein drink if you
want to.

Here is how I generally make my protein drink. Using whey protein
from the health food store, I mix it as follows: 20 grams protein, 10 fro-
zen strawberries, 2 tablespoons spirulina, 1 cup sugar-free lemonade
or lite juice, 4 Splenda packets (xylitol or agave nectar are the organic
versions of sugar-free sweeteners), and a dash of cinnamon. Put all of
these ingredients into a blender and mix until smooth. I have this protein shake every morning, along with my vitamins.

I listed protein foods first in the shopping list because I believe they
are the most significant way you can stabilize your energy, even out
your moods, and reduce cravings. Whenever possible, choose low-fat,
organic versions of these foods. Eat a minimum of 60 grams of protein

daily, preferably in 10- to 20-gram servings spaced evenly throughout the day. If you are exercising or working out frequently, you'll need twice as much protein to compensate. To continue our shopping list:

Our Shopping List of Vegetables, Fruits, and Desserts

Vegetables	Fruits	Desserts
Lettuce/spinach	Apples	Russell Stover sugar-free candy (see below)
Zucchini	Oranges	Toffee
Tomatoes	All berries	Truffles
Eggplant	Plums	Hard candies
Onions	Pears	Caramels
Mushrooms	Melons	Pecan clusters
Bell peppers	Grapefruit	Sugar-free ice cream
Carrots	Peaches	Sugar-free pudding
Cucumber	Grapes	Sugar-free hot cocoa
Broccoli	Etc.	Most desserts can be made in low-fat, sugar-free, and/or wheat-free versions
Asparagus		
Etc.		

Really, all vegetables and fruits are fine as long as they're fresh, preferably organic, and you don't overdo it on the starchy ones like dried fruits, bananas, yams, potatoes, and corn.

Does the dessert category have your tastebuds humming? As I've said, I don't believe in deprivation. I've created excellent versions of sugar-free pumpkin custard, rice pudding, fruit pudding, cheesecake, stewed fruit over sugar-free vanilla ice cream, and other treats. If there is a way to enjoy some of the sweet tastes and textures *without setting off any triggers to overeat,* I believe it's fine to have dessert—in moderation! Unfortunately, some people find that even the no-sugar versions of these treats will tempt them into overeating. As I've said, you will need to experiment to see what works for you and what doesn't.

Note: Some sugar-free sweeteners will give you diarrhea if you eat more than two or three servings at a sitting (one piece of candy is considered a serving). You've been warned!

Back to the shopping list:

Our Shopping List of Fats, Oils, and Beverages

Fats and oils	Beverages
Extra-virgin olive oil	Water
Flaxseed oil	Sugar-free fruit drinks
Other EFA oils (e.g., fish oil)	Teas
Butter	Coffee (preferably decaf)
Coconut oil	Sugar-free sodas (avoid sodas that are very fizzy if you're a new WLS post-op)
Sesame oil	Juice

EFA oils (flaxseed oil, fish oils) can't be cooked with; instead, add a couple of teaspoons to your salad dressing, or take them as a supplement in capsule form. However and whenever you use oils, always use the least amount necessary.

Fresh, organic fruit juices (the kind with no added sugar) are very nutritious, but even they are a very concentrated source of naturally occurring sugar. Try a blend of half juice, half sparkling water or club soda (or one-third juice, two-thirds sparkling water).

Beverages with aspartame or caffeine should be avoided or consumed sparingly. Sugar-free sweeteners are an ongoing controversy. The healthier ones, like stevia, agave nectar, or birch bark (xylitol), have an unusual taste that goes with some foods but not others. The chemical versions, like Splenda (sucralose), Equal (aspartame), and

Sweet'N Low (saccharin), taste better to some people but aren't so healthy. Anything ending in "-ose" (e.g., fructose, glucose, sucrose) is a sugar. Anything ending in "-ol" (e.g., malitol, sorbitol, xylitol) doesn't taste bad but tends to give you the runs if you eat too much of it. There's no perfect solution. I use Splenda in some things, stevia or xylitol in others, cooked raisins in others.

You may have noticed that I haven't listed any traditional high-carbohydrate foods such as bread, pasta, bagels, and the like. This is because many chronic overeaters, including me, suffer from an allergic/addicted response to these foods (which triggers monster cravings for more), even complex carbs or whole-wheat varieties. Some people even have this sort of reaction to most or all grain-based foods, not just wheat. Your body will tell you whether or not you can safely eat them. If you are unsure about your reaction, you can try the healthier, whole-grain versions and see how you feel when you eat them. If you tend to binge on them, you can try the excellent alternative pastas, breads, and flour that are made from grains such as spelt, rice, oat flour, garbanzo flour, tapioca, quinoa, or amaranth, all of which are available at natural-foods stores. Sadly, I found that even these foods were triggers for me, so I eat them very rarely. For you, they may be fine. Listen to your body and see what foods leave you feeling energized and clear and which ones leave you feeling fogged, tired, and craving more food than you need.

Also, remember that if you write down your food plan, you'll be much more likely to stick to it. I wrote mine daily before and after surgery, and I still do if I get off track. It helps!

Amino Acid Therapy

A cautionary suggestion: Please educate yourself thoroughly and check with your doctor before trying amino acid therapy. If your best determination to stick to a food plan often gets sidetracked by cravings, try using specific amino acids to combat this problem. L-glutamine, which regulates blood sugar, is very helpful in preventing cravings. (All the aminos work best on an empty stomach, so take them either twenty minutes before or ninety minutes after a meal. Also, it is good to take the supplements at the times when you are usually tempted to overeat.) Consult the chart on the next page, which is from Julia Ross's book *The Diet Cure,* to determine which other aminos will help you. I use DL-Phenylalanine (DLPA) and 5-HTP. The general dosage for each of these is as follows:

- L-Tyrosine: 500–1,500 mg (2–3 times a day)
- GABA: 100–500 mg (1–3 times a day)
- DL-Phenylalanine (DLPA): 500–1,500 mg (2–3 times a day)
- L-Tryptophan/5-HTP: 50–150mg (2–3 times a day)
- Melatonin: 500–1,500 mg (2–3 times a day)
- L-Glutamine: 500–1,500 (2–3 times a day)

These dosages are explained in detail in *The Diet Cure,* and I highly encourage you to read the book for more specific information on this subject.

Here's a summary of which amino acids are effective for treating certain conditions associated with food cravings:

- If you frequently feel emotionally overwhelmed and you tend to be overstressed and high-strung, tense, and unable to relax, try GABA.
- If you crave food for comfort or to numb overly sensitive feelings, try DLPA.
- If you have a negative outlook; are worried, anxious, and depressed; and typically get evening cravings, try 5-HTP.
- If you are often sluggish and have a hard time concentrating or getting up in the morning, try L-tyrosine (and have your thyroid function checked).
- If you have insomnia, try melatonin.

○ If you have big peaks and valleys in your energy and blood-sugar levels, try L-glutamine.

Many of my clients were so excited by this information that they ran out and bought all the amino acids at once or formulas that combine all twenty-two amino acids into one supplement. Doing this doesn't work, at least not for the symptoms listed above. I encourage you to try them one at a time to determine which ones have the most positive effect on you. This way, you won't waste money or time taking several at once and then wonder which one made you feel better!

Amino Acid Therapy Chart

Neuro-transmitter	Promotes	Deficiency results in	Drugs that affect	Amino acids needed
Norepi-nephrine	Arousal, energy, drive, mental focus	Lack of drive, depression, lack of energy, lack of focus, ADD (Attention Deficit Disorder)	Sugar, chocolate, caffeine, cocaine, amphetamines, tobacco, marijuana, alcohol, aspartame	L-Tyrosine
GABA	Staying calm, relaxation	Tension, stress, inability to relax, feeling overwhelmed	Carbs, Valium, marijuana, tobacco, alcohol	GABA
Endorphins	Psychological and physical pain relief, comfort, pleasure, reward, loving feelings	Overly sensitive to emotional and physical pain, cries easily, seeks pleasure, comfort, reward, numbness	Chocolate, marijuana, alcohol, sugar, starch, tobacco, heroin	DL-Phenylalanine (DLPA)

(cont'd.)

Amino Acid Therapy Chart (cont'd.)

Neuro-transmitter	Promotes	Deficiency results in	Drugs that affect	Amino acids needed
Serotonin	Positive ("sunny") disposition, emotional stability, self-confidence	Negativity, anxiety, irritability, obsession, worry, panic, low self-esteem, PMS, evening cravings, winter depression, heat intolerance	Sugar, starch, marijuana, ecstasy, tobacco, alcohol, Prozac	L-Tryptophan, or 5 HTP (5-Hydroxy-tryptophan) (Exercise) (Light therapy)
(Melatonin)	Optimal sleep	Sleep problems		Melatonin
Brain fuel (glucose)	Stable blood sugar	Cravings for alcohol, sugar, starch	Alcohol, sugar, starch	L-Glutamine

Reprinted courtesy of Julia Ross

A Daily Food Plan in Action*

* Please note that for gastric bypass patients, the portions suggested here are for one year post-op and thereafter.

Three meals and two snacks work well for most people. Here's a sample:

7:30 A.M. — 6–10 oz. light juice or water, with your amino acids (e.g., DLPA, L-glutamine, and/or L-Tyrosine).

Breakfast (8 A.M.) — Two-egg omelet, with ½ c. sautéed veggies and 2 oz. cheese; or an 8–10 oz. protein drink with fruit, 20 grams protein powder, light juice, or low-fat milk (add stevia or Splenda if you want it sweeter). Either just before or right after breakfast, be sure to take your vitamins with plenty of water, and any other supplements that are supposed to be taken with food.

Snack (10 or 10:30 A.M.) — 2 oz. cheese w/an apple, or 6 oz. sugar-free yogurt with fruit, or a handful of nuts/raisins.

Lunch (12:30 or 1 P.M.) — Cobb salad: 1–2 c. lettuce, ¼ avocado, 2 oz. deli meats, 2 oz. cheese, 1 boiled egg. A great dressing is 1 tablespoon balsamic vinegar and 1–2 tablespoons EFA oil.

Or, make a quick a stir-fry with 3–4 oz. protein (e.g., tofu, fish, chicken, pork, beans) and 1–2 cups sliced veggies. I steam the veggies first so they won't need much oil. (Microwave method for steaming: Put cut veggies into a plastic bag with a little water, and cook on high for 2–3 minutes.) Sauté the protein in 1–2 tablespoons sesame oil or olive oil, add the veggies, soy sauce to taste, ½ teaspoon ginger powder, and 1 Splenda packet.

2:30 P.M. — Time for more amino acids, especially if this is the time of day when you would normally be tired and indulge in some kind of pick-me-up like coffee or sweets. L-tyrosine or DLPA (500–1,500 mg) can provide a good source of natural energy. Along with L-Glutamine or 5-HTP they can knock out cravings, too.

Snack (3 P.M.) — Same as the morning snack, or have 2–3 oz. protein and a small portion of fruit or veggies.

Dinner (6 or 7 P.M.) — 4–5 oz. protein, 1–2 cups steamed veggies, and a salad provides a good basic framework. Try pan-seared salmon (using 1–2 tablespoons butter or olive oil) with a lemon-dill seasoning; steamed asparagus with 1 teaspoon butter; and a green salad with 2 oz. feta cheese, 1 tomato, ½ cucumber, ¼ red onion, and a few olives and artichoke hearts. Use the same salad dressing as above. Sound yummy? It is.

To stop evening cravings and get you to sleep, 5-HTP and/or melatonin can be really effective.

Snack (8 or 9 P.M.) — Here is where I break away from most diets you'll ever see. I don't believe in feeling deprived, and if you tell me I can't have a nighttime snack, sooner or later I'll rebel. I do allow myself this treat, within reason. I'll enjoy a cup of sugar-free cocoa with a little added milk, or a sugar-free candy, or a cut-up steamed apple with Splenda and cinnamon, or a cup of decaf or herbal tea.

How to Really Enjoy Exercise

The next phase is to get the body moving. Remember, our body is our friend and it needs to move! What if you had a dog that you never took for a walk? You'd know you were depriving your pet of a much-needed part of its overall health and enjoyment. The same thing goes for your body. I think the reason we often feel resistance at the idea of moving the body is because we call it *exercise* and make it torturous. There is absolutely no reason to do this to yourself! If you love the gym, great, go for it. I prefer swimming, hiking, gardening, horseback riding, backpacking—something that gets me outside, either with friends or with my dog. Then I really enjoy moving, rather than either avoiding it or dragging myself through it.

Lifting weights can be very helpful. Pound for pound, muscle burns more calories than other types of body tissue, even when you are at rest. If you can find a place in your heart and your lifestyle for weightlifting, great. If not, that's okay too. Many forms of exercise (e.g., swimming, dancing, hiking, cycling) build moderate amounts of muscle.

The minimum amount of physical activity recommended by most health experts is half an hour of vigorous movement at least three times a week (but preferably five times a week), to the point where you are panting, or, hopefully, panting and sweating. Come on now, there were times when panting and sweating were a lot of fun, right?

Many of us have spent our whole lives disassociated from our bodies—that is, feeling as if we live only in our head, or only in our relationship to the outside world, never really *in* our body. It's easy to understand this disassociation when you consider that many of us have felt at war with our bodies, like our bodies were resisting and defying our attempts at improvement. We wanted them to look a certain way— but they didn't. We wanted them to lose weight—but they wouldn't. We wanted them to look good to other people, make us desirable, or at least allow us to be fashionable—but the response we wanted from others didn't happen. No wonder we pretended our bodies weren't really a part of us! Add health problems to this equation, and the war escalated. One of the biggest mental, emotional, and spiritual shifts I hope you'll make is realizing that *you can't hate your body and love yourself at the same time.*

Also, consider that this is the only body you've got, and it will be with you your whole life. Do you really want to end up being one of those old people who go on endlessly about their ailments? Regular exercise is one of the surest ways to keep yourself fit and healthy over the long haul. It's worth it, and once you get into the groove, you'll find yourself actually craving it. It's your body that craves movement.

There are many ways to get back in touch with your body—yoga, deep breathing, dancing, massage, even lovemaking or sensual touch if you have a partner whom you trust. Make friends with your body, and you'll be surprised at how much more content and centered you will feel.

Things to Do Besides Eat When You're Not Really Hungry

◎

Finally, here is a list of fun activities, developed by my OEE support group, to refer to in those restless moments when you want to eat:

— Go to the beach   — Watch the sunset
— Work out   — Help out in your community
— Watch TV   — Get/give hugs
— Draw a picture   — Clean a closet

— Meditate
— Go window-shopping
— Do some gardening
— Do crafts/hobbies
— Just be
— Cook healthy food
— Play a musical instrument
— Exercise
— Listen to the birds sing
— Read
— Do volunteer work
— Go swimming
— Journal
— Float in the ocean
— Pet a pet
— Go to a meeting
— Nurture yourself
— Try something new
— Practice forgiveness
— Drink water
— Get support
— Go for a drive
— Watch a movie
— Spend time with loved ones
— Go to the park
— Decorate something
— Write about "What do I *really* want?"

— Pray
— Play with animals
— Sing
— Share with a friend
— Listen to music
— Just feel it
— Dance
— Light candles
— Make a photo album
— Read a self-help book
— Trust your spirit
— Make love
— Play with kids
— Go hiking
— Just breathe deeply for 10 minutes
— Get into counseling
— Talk it out
— Have a of cup tea
— Love yourself
— Lie in the sun
— Give support
— Surf the Internet
— Get affection
— Go for a walk
— Plant flowers
— Create something beautiful

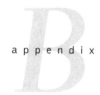

appendix

How to Start Your Own Support Group

Support groups are wonderful resources for helping people find the strength, humor, and wisdom to follow a food and exercise plan. If you live in an area that doesn't have a support group for people dealing with chronic overeating, don't give up. You can start one! Even if you begin the group by yourself, before long it will be rolling along on its own. Whether you are a WLS post-op wanting to stay on track, or an overeater trying to get on track, having the support of your peers is invaluable.

Here are the steps to take to start a group:

1. Decide on a focus for the group. Will it be freedom from compulsive eating? Will it be a place to vent your emotions and cheer each other forward? Will you follow a workbook and do assignments as a group?

2. Once you're clear on your focus, you'll need to advertise for participants. Your local newspaper, especially a small weekly paper, should be an effective way to do so. Here's a sample ad: "Support group now forming to discuss healthy eating/weight

loss. Help yourself and others to become the person you've always wanted to be, free from excess pounds and food cravings. First meeting on [date]. Confidential, no fee. Call [phone number]."

3. If you are going to use a book or workbook, specify which one so members can look it over before attending the first meeting. Of course, I think *this* book would be a good choice, especially since all of the assignments evolved from my work with support groups.

4. Hold an initial meeting to decide on the following issues:
   o Best place to hold your ongoing meetings.
   o Will you meet weekly, biweekly, or monthly?
   o How long will each meeting be? (Hint: Ninety minutes.)
   o To cover incidental expenses, will you take a donation? Charge a fee?
   o Will your group be closed (i.e., no new members after a certain point) or open?
   o Will you allow food or drink at the meetings?
   o Will you allow those with other active addictions, like alcoholism or drug addiction, to attend?
   o Will it be coed, or open to only one gender?
   o Will you allow kids or family members to be present, even if they just want to check it out? (Hint: No.)
   o Will you allow group members to go on and on, or will there be a suggested time limit for each person's sharing? (Hint: Three to five minutes each.)
   o Will you allow "cross-talk," i.e., interrupting, advice-giving, one member focusing more on someone else's sharing than on his/her own issues? (Hint: No way!)
   o Will you have one person run the meeting? Will this job rotate? How long will each person hold the job?

o Will you decide on a set of guidelines for, say, three months, then reevaluate how well it's working?

Once you make these decisions, it's also crucial to discuss how to keep your group a safe and inspiring place for all. Privacy concerns, basic courtesy concerns, too-frequent negative whining instead of being solution-oriented—all these issues can make or break a group.

If starting a support group seems like more than you are ready for, consider checking out a group such as Weight Watchers, Overeaters Anonymous, Food Addicts Anonymous, or T.O.P.S., all of which are available nationwide (see the Resources section for contact information).

You can also find support groups and chat groups online. Yahoo Groups lists over *nine hundred* such groups for people who have been through weight loss surgery. To reach them, go to the website groups. yahoo.com, type "weight loss surgery" into the search box—and there you are! You'll have lots and lots of choices for chat rooms, support, information, and links to other helpful sites on WLS.

Resources

Helpful Websites

OA: www.overeatersanonymous.com

Weight Watchers: www.weightwatchers.com

FAA: www.foodaddictsanonymous.org

T.O.P.S. (Take Off Pounds Sensibly): www.tops.com

Another useful weight loss site: www.sparkpeople.com

If you are interested in chat group–style online support, Yahoo sponsors over nine hundred groups on weight loss surgery and related topics. To access them, visit the website groups.yahoo.com, and type in "weight loss surgery."

WLS Information Sites

www.obesityhelp.com

www.weightlosssurgeryoptions.com

www.onpointhealth.com

www.wlscenter.com

www.wfubmc.edu

www.pbs.org (Under "Programs A–Z" click on *Frontline,* then search for "weight loss surgery")

www.nlm.nih.gov

Books

On Learning Healthy Eating Habits

The Diet Cure by Julia Ross

Eating in the Light of the Moon by Anita Johnston

Making Peace with Food by Susan Kano

Lighten Up Your Body, Lighten Up Your Life by Lucia Cappacione

Abstinence in Action by Barbara McFarland and Anne Marie Erb

The Only Diet There Is by Sondra Ray

Feeding the Hungry Heart by Geneen Roth

Breaking Free from Compulsive Eating by Geneen Roth

Intuitive Eating by Evelyn Tribole and Elyse Resch

Passing For Thin by Frances Kuffel

The Twelve Steps of Overeaters Anonymous

Overeaters Anonymous (or any of OA's literature, available at www.overeatersanonymous.com)

On Relationships and Codependency

Codependent No More by Melody Beattie

Beyond Codependency by Melody Beattie

A Codependent's Guide to the Twelve Steps by Melody Beattie

Healing the Shame That Binds You by John Bradshaw

Bradshaw On: The Family by John Bradshaw

Codependents Anonymous

On Inner Child Work

Homecoming: Reclaiming and Championing Your Inner Child by John Bradshaw

Self-Parenting by Mark Lucas

Recovery of Your Inner Child by Lucia Cappacione

Author Contact Information

To contact the author, ask for an Overcoming Emotional Eating seminar in your area, or order copies of this book or the accompanying
workbook for groups, please write or e-mail Michelle Ritchie at the
following address:

Michelle Ritchie
1120 Maohu St.
Makawao HI 96768
E-mail: mlrmaui@yahoo.com

Index